D0061462

MOTOR SPEECH DISORDERS

Diagnosis and Treatment

DONALD B. FREED, Ph.D.
California State University, Fresno

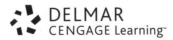

DELMAR
CENGAGE Learning

Australia • Canada • Mexico • Singapore • Spain • United Kingdom • United States

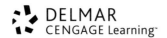

Motor Speech Disorders
Diagnosis and Treatment
Donald B. Freed, Ph.D.

For product information and technology assistance, contact us at
Cengage Learning Customer & Sales Support, 1-800-354-9706

For permission to use material from this text or product,
submit all requests online at **cengage.com/permissions**
Further permissions questions can be emailed to

Library of Congress Control Number: 99038078

ISBN-13: 978-1-56593-951-6

ISBN-10: 1-56593-951-4

Delmar Cengage Learning
5 Maxwell Drive
Clifton Park, NY 12065-2919
USA

Cengage Learning products are represented in Canada by Nelson Education, Ltd.

For your lifelong learning solutions, visit
delmar.cengage.com

Visit our corporate website at **www.cengage.com**

Notice to the Reader
Publisher does not warrant or guarantee any of the products described herein or perform any independent analysis in connection with any of the product information contained herein. Publisher does not assume, and expressly disclaims, any obligation to obtain and include information other than that provided to it by the manufacturer. The reader is expressly warned to consider and adopt all safety precautions that might be indicated by the activities described herein and to avoid all potential hazards. By following the instructions contained herein, the reader willingly assumes all risks in connection with such instructions. The publisher makes no representations or warranties of any kind, including but not limited to, the warranties of fitness for particular purpose or merchantability, nor are any such representations implied with respect to the material set forth herein, and the publisher takes no responsibility with respect to such material. The publisher shall not be liable for any special, consequential, or exemplary damages resulting, in whole or part, from the readers' use of, or reliance upon, this material.

Printed in Canada
11 12 13 14 13 12 11 10 09

Contents

Preface

This book was written with graduate students and beginning speech-language pathologists in mind. The author knows from his own graduate school experience how confusing and complicated motor speech disorders can be. Even the best students (and instructors) can find it difficult to grasp the many neurological and clinical aspects of these disorders. The overall goal of this book is to present the topic of motor speech disorders in the most clear, uncluttered manner possible. This has been a challenging task because of the complexity of the subject matter. Motor speech disorders involve some of the most complex parts of the nervous system. They also are very wide-ranging in their etiologies, symptoms, and treatments. Deciding what to include and exclude from this book was similar to walking a tightrope. On one side, enough detail had to be included to fully describe the disorders. On the other side, certain details were omitted so as to keep the reader from being overwhelmed with too many facts about anatomy, neurology, and so forth.

In trying to present this topic as clearly as possible, it was necessary to repeat certain facts about these disorders in various parts of the book. For example, the function of the cerebellum is discussed first in Chapter 3 (The Motor System), and it is reviewed again in Chapter 7 (Ataxic Dysarthria). The same can be said for the neurological basis of spastic dysarthria, which appears in numerous parts of the text. This type of repetition is most evident in the repeated listings of certain treatment procedures in different chapters. These listings are repeated because early in the development of this book, it was decided to include the treatment suggestions for each specific disorder within the chapter discussing that disorder, rather than the more traditional method of presenting all treatment procedures in a separate chapter. With this type of organization, each chapter presents the entire clinical picture of a specific motor speech disorder, from its etiology to its treatment. However, because numerous treatment procedures are appropriate for more than one motor speech disorder, some repetition from chapter to chapter was inevitable.

The overall organization of the book is straightforward. Chapter 1 is a review of very early case reports that seem to involve speech or language disorders. It is designed as a historical introduction to the study of motor speech disorders. Chapter 2 discusses how speech-language pathologists evaluate these disorders. A major portion of this chapter is a step-by-step explanation of a detailed motor speech protocol. It explains what each assessment task examines and why it is significant. Chapter 3 is an introduction to the human motor system, certainly one of the most marvelous and complicated parts of the nervous system. As mentioned in that chapter, it is essential that clinicians have at least a basic understanding of the motor system if they are going to accurately diagnose and treat motor speech disorders. The remainder of the book, Chapters 4 through 11, covers the six pure dysarthrias, mixed dysarthria, and apraxia of speech. Throughout these chapters, a consistent organization has been maintained, so as to facilitate the reader's understanding of the disorders. Each begins with the neurological basis of the condition, then continues with the etiologies of the disorder, a survey of the relevant speech characteristics, key evaluation tasks specific to the disorder, and concludes with treatment suggestions.

Acknowledgments

Many friends and colleagues helped complete this book. Dr. Giri Hegde had the confidence to ask me to write it. He also served as one of the reviewers for the first draft of the manuscript. Dee Garvin and Teryl Gough both were excellent student assistants and did much of the essential (but unexciting) collecting of basic information. Carl Knox did nearly all of the technical work on the CD-ROM. It certainly would not have possible to put the videos to computer disk without his extraordinary expertise. It was a pleasure working with the folks at Singular Publishing. Their many gentle yet firm questions about when various chapters would be completed were an invaluable part of getting the work done. Lastly, sincere thanks must go the patients who appear on the CD-ROM. Each of them generously donated his or her time and effort to the videotapings. If anything, I hope the book and CD-ROM is a tribute to their spirit and determination to lead normal lives.

Dedication

To Jean and Clyde
for being great parents
and to
Adrian, Cassandra, MacLean, and Rowan

C H A P T E R

1

A Brief Historical Review of Motor Speech Disorders

A. Case Reports From Ancient Greece
B. Case Reports From The Middle Ages and Renaissance
C. Two Early Theories on the Localization of Reason
D. From the 19th Century to Today

The term *motor speech disorders* is an apt description of the deficits that are examined in this textbook. To help readers who are new to the study of motor speech disorders, it will be beneficial to discuss the meaning of each word in this term. First of all, *motor* is the part of the nervous system that controls voluntary movements. Neuroanatomists call this portion of the nervous system the motor system. *Speech*, of course, is communication through the use of vocal symbols, sometimes also defined as the physical production of language. *Disorders* means an abnormality of function, and because the word is plural, it indicates that there is more than one abnormality in this condition. Motor speech disorders, therefore, are a collection of speech production deficits that are caused by the abnormal functioning of the motor system. Altogether, this collection of motor speech disorders consists of seven types of dysarthria and one type of apraxia.

Although the following chapters contain detailed discussions of dysarthria and apraxia, these disorders need to be briefly defined now. The literal definition of *dysarthria* is disordered utterance (*dys* means disordered or abnormal; *arthria* means to utter distinctly, from the Greek, *arthroun*). A more comprehensive definition is that dysarthria is the impaired production of speech because of disturbances in the muscular control of the speech mechanism. The layperson's concept of dysarthria is someone who has slurred speech, but this disorder certainly includes many more speech production deficits than just poor articulation. It can involve respiration, prosody, resonance, and phonation as well.

Apraxia of speech also is a motor speech disorder. *Apraxia* means without action (*a* means absence of; *praxia* means performance of action, from the Greek, *praxis*). Actually, apraxia of speech is a deficit in the ability to smoothly sequence the speech producing movements of the tongue, lips, jaw, and so forth. Apraxia of speech primarily affects articulation and prosody. Although apraxia of speech occurs frequently when the left hemisphere of the brain is damaged, the general public seems to be less aware of the characteristics of this disorder than they are of dysarthria.

Before moving to the clinical aspects of motor speech disorders, this chapter reviews a small selection of ancient medical reports that mention speech and language disorders. It is important to examine these early reports, because a valuable part of any study is understanding the historical context from which the subject developed. Whether the topic is science or entertainment, a historical perspective adds a sense of depth and continuity that is otherwise difficult to obtain. While reading the following pages, keep in mind that some of the individuals in these case studies experienced their speech and language disorders more than 2,000 years ago.

One of the most remarkable aspects of preparing this chapter was the discovery of how "modern" many of these ancient medical writers were. From today's perspective, it is easy to view them as quaint at best or frightfully ignorant at worst. But when examined in the context in which they lived, these physicians' conclusions about anatomy and physiology show that most of them were trying to take an analytical approach to medicine. When reading their descriptions of their medical practice, it is easy to imagine them as today's state-of-the-art practitioners. Their writings show that many of them were actively seeking a more complete understanding of the human body and were trying to find better ways of treating their patients. Although these early physicians were wrong about many details, their writings reveal that they were attempting to be reasonable and thoughtful professionals.

CASE REPORTS FROM ANCIENT GREECE

Some of the earliest written accounts of speech and language disorders appear in the Greek texts known as the Hippocratic Corpus. Originally, these texts were a collection of 70 volumes that described numerous medicines, diseases, and treatments, as observed by ancient Greek physicians. Only about 60 of these volumes survive to the present, but the remaining works contain many descriptions of anatomy, explanations of symptoms, and case studies of patients. A sampling of the individual titles gives an idea of the wide-ranging topics covered in these works. The titles include "On Ancient Medicines," "On Fractures," "The Book of Prognostics," and "Of the Epidemics." There are even volumes devoted to ulcers and hemorrhoids. Some of these works were written for educated physicians and contain surprising amounts of specific information about medical disorders and how to treat them. Other volumes were written for the general public and are, accordingly, more plainspoken in their advice.

The authorship of the Hippocratic Corpus is a bit of a mystery. Although it carries his name, Hippocrates (460?–?377 BC) was not the sole writer of this collection (Figure 1–1). In fact, it is not certain that he wrote any of the volumes. Most experts believe that numerous writers contributed to the collection during a period of at least 100 years. It is possible that the actual writers were physicians who were part of a school founded by Hippocrates on the Greek island of Kos.

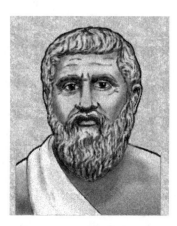

Figure 1–1. An artist's representation of Hippocrates (460?–?377 BC), who may or may not have contributed to the ancient medical texts that carry his name.

Among the many descriptions of disorders in the Hippocratic Corpus are numerous references to patients being "speechless" or having "loss of speech." A few of these seem to be references to neurologically based speech or language disorders. For example, in Book One in "Of the Epidemics" (circa 400 BC), there is a description of what could be an instance of aphasia and right hemiplegia.

> A woman, who lodged on the Quay, being three months gone with child, was seized with fever, and immediately began to have pains in the loins. On the third day, pain of the head and neck, extending to the clavicle, and right hand; she immediately lost the power of speech; was paralyzed in the right hand, with spasms, after the manner of paraplegia; was quite incoherent; passed an uncomfortable night. ("Of the Epidemics" [400 BC/1995])

Fortunately, the woman's speech or language deficit, whatever it might have been, was only temporary because on the next day, she "recovered the use of her tongue," and on the sixth day, she "recovered her reason."

Another volume in the Hippocratic Corpus contains descriptions that also may be references to neurologically based speech or language disorders. In the "Aphorisms" (400 BC/1995), the writer makes an intriguing comment about the rapid onset of a condition that is accompanied by speechlessness. "When persons in good health are suddenly seized with pains in the head, and straightway are laid down speechless, and breathe with stertor, they die in seven days, unless fever comes on." Although it is impossible to determine with certainty, this may be a description of the sudden onset of a stroke or some other neurological disorder. Garrison (1925/1969) suggested that this passage describes a subarachnoid hemorrhage, a condition that is nearly always accompanied by a sudden, painful headache and the rapid onset of other neurological signs. A second intriguing comment from the "Aphorisms" seems to be a reference to the loss of speech after a head injury, "In cases of concussion of the brain produced by any cause, the patients necessarily lose their speech." As with the prior quote, it is difficult to determine which modern day condition this may be describing. It could be that the loss of speech is the result of aphasia, severe dysarthria, or merely a temporary loss of consciousness.

One of the more detailed accounts of head injury resulting in a speech or language deficit is found in Book Five of *Of the Epidemics*. It describes what happened to a young woman who was playing with a friend.

> The pretty virgin daughter of Nerius was twenty years old. She was struck on the *bregma* (front of the head) by the flat of the hand of a young woman friend in play. At the time she became blind and breathless, and when she went home fever seized her immediately, her head ached, and there was redness about her face. On the seventh day foul-smelling pus came out around the right ear, reddish, more than a cyathus (one-fifth of a cup). She seemed better, and was relieved. Again she was prostrated by the fever; she was depressed, speechless; the right side of her face was drawn up; she had difficulty breathing; there was a spasmodic trembling. Her tongue was paralyzed, her eye stricken. On the ninth day she died. (Smith, 1994, p. 191)

This description indicates clearly that the author believed that the cause of the woman's speechlessness was the blow to her head. However, the type of speech or language disorder she had is difficult to determine. A modern day reader might assume that dysarthria was a part of the problem because of the reference to a paralyzed tongue and facial contractions, but this conclusion would be little more than conjecture.

Numerous examples of disordered voice are found in Book Seven of *Of the Epidemics*. One of the more intriguing reports described a woman with arthritis whose "voice was checked during the night and up to midday." Although she could not talk, "she could hear, her mind was clear; she indicated with her hand that the pain was around the hip joint" (Smith, 1994, p. 399). That her auditory comprehension was functional and that she could gesture appropriately suggests that her speechlessness was from a laryngeal disorder, although it is difficult to say with certainty. Another case report tells of a man in Olynthus who had a "fever" for 17 days. The writer described him as having a "dreadful disorganization of body" and that his "voice [was] broken, a task to hear it, but intelligible" (Smith, 1994, p. 377). Once again, the author's imprecise description of the man's deficits make it difficult to know what was wrong with his speech or voice. The man might have been demonstrating the effects of a neurological speech impairment such as dysarthria or, perhaps, his voice was only soft and breathy from his weakened condition.

All of these case studies from the Hippocratic Corpus show that the ancient Greeks understood that speech difficulties could be the result of physical injury. Most important, these writings indicate that the Greeks understood that injury to the head could cause speechlessness (O'Neill, 1980). It is less certain whether they had a modern day understanding of how voice, speech, and language differ, as can be seen in their vague medical descriptions of these communicative processes. Nevertheless, the influence of the Hippocratic Corpus on Western medicine was long lasting. It was part of the standard medical curriculum for nearly 2,000 years. As late as the 18th century, some physicians were still studying and practicing the Hippocratic teachings on medicine.

CASE REPORTS FROM THE MIDDLE AGES AND RENAISSANCE

Early descriptions of speech and language disorders did not end with the Greeks. Medical texts from the Middle Ages and Renaissance also provide various examples of these problems. For instance, in the early 1300s, a physician named Bernard of Gordon described individuals who omitted and added syllables to their speech (O'Neill, 1980). His examples of their spoken words (e.g., saying Aristoles for Aristoteles) are intriguing and have characteristics that are similar to those in apraxia of speech. But as with the case studies from the Hippocratic Corpus, the exact natures of the patients' disorders cannot be determined from the writer's descriptions of their speech.

Another example of a speech or language disorder from the medieval era comes from an Italian physician, Lanfranc. He wrote about an incident in which a man fell from a horse and injured his head. After regaining consciousness, the man's initial attempts at speech were filled with what Lanfranc described as a child's babble—something that today might be labeled neologistic jargon or perhaps the language of confusion. The man did survive the accident, and his speech eventually became intelligible. Unfortunately the recovery was not complete, because Lanfranc reported that the man never recovered the full faculties of his mind.

In the mid-1500s, a physician named Niccolo Massa recorded the details of another head injury that resulted in disordered speech. His case report is of a young man who was hit in the head with a spear, which apparently pierced deeply into his skull.

> Also returned to health by my work is the noble youth, Marcus Goro who was wounded by the sharp point of a spear . . . . There was fracture of not only the cranial bone, but of the meninges, and of the brain substance as far as to the basilar bone . . . . Besides all his other difficulties, the young man had been speechless for eight days . . . . Since the physicians declared they had seen no bone, I thought that the reason for the extinction of the voice was that there was a piece of bone fixed in the brain, and taking an instrument from a certain surgeon who was there, I extracted the bone from the wound, and immediately, he began to speak, and said, "Praise God, I am healed." (O'Neill, 1980, p. 185)

TWO EARLY THEORIES ON THE LOCALIZATION OF REASON

Early medical writings were not confined to case reports of injuries. Many of them also included the author's thoughts on how the human body functioned. Some of the most interesting of these are the theories of where human reasoning (and by implication, speech and language) was located in the body. One of the most long-lasting theories stated that reasoning was housed in the four cerebral ventricles. It was thought that the two lateral ventricles were where the body received sensory information from the outside world. This sensory information was believed to be then moved to the third ventricle, which contained the intellect. It was thought that the intellect analyzed the information and extracted meaning from sensory information. The fourth ventricle was believed to be responsible for memory—storing sensory information once it had been analyzed.

Evidence for this theory was described by such writers as Galen (130?–?200 BC), who observed that the closer a wound was to the ventricles, the more serious were the consequences for the patient. For instance, a surface wound to the brain usually did not result in deficits that were as significant as a wound that penetrated deeply into cerebral tissue. Because the deeper wound caused more serious damage and was closer to the ventricles, it was hypothesized that the ventricles must play an important role in cognitive abilities. Although this theory of ventricular localization was incorrect, it was nevertheless nearer the truth than an earlier theory that placed the centers for speech and emotion in the heart. The ventricle hypothesis was an enduring one. It lasted from ancient times to the 16th century. This theory also had many noted followers, such as Leonardo da Vinci (1452–1519) who included the ventricles in many of his anatomical drawings of the nervous system (Figure 1–2). It finally was discredited when Vesalius (1514–1564) reasoned that because the cerebral ventricles in animals' brains were so similar in shape and number to those in human brains, it was unlikely that the ventricles played an especially important part in human reasoning.

A second, contemporaneous theory about the center for human reasoning held that the senses and movement were controlled by the meninges, which are the membranes that cover the brain and spinal cord. In brief, this theory was based on the observation that whenever the meninges were damaged by an injury, there almost always was some deficit in a patient's reasoning abilities, whether it was memory, movement, sensation, speech, or some other mental faculty. The wide acceptance of this theory is reflected by the fact that many early case studies of head injury frequently mentioned whether there was damage to the meninges, as seen in the prior quote from Massa. Another example of this can be found in a 1514 medical text by Giovanni da Vigo. He described a nobleman who was seriously injured when he fell from a horse and was kicked in the head. The man's subsequent speechlessness was attributed to sharp bone fragments that had pierced his meninges. No mention was made that the fragments might have damaged the underlying brain tissue. The meningeal theory was accepted widely for many centuries. Some physicians were still ascribing to it as late as the 16th century (O'Neill, 1980).

FROM THE 19TH CENTURY TO TODAY

Before the 19th century, most descriptions of speech and language disorders were too vague to be identified as definite historical instances

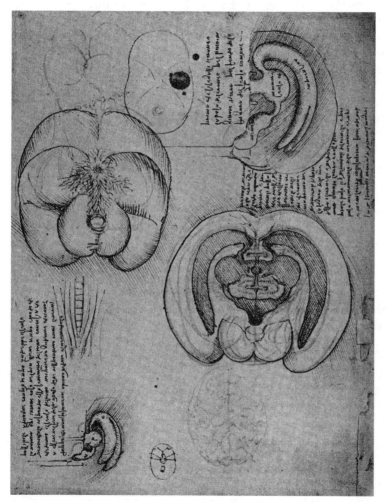

Figure 1–2. Leonardo da Vinci (1452–1519) believed that the cerebral ventricles were the containers of human intellect and featured them prominently in many of his anatomical drawings. This drawing is almost certainly of an ox's brain.

of motor speech disorders. Reports that seemed to describe a motor speech disorder had to remain intriguing possibilities, because they were lacking in detail. This began to change in the early 1800s, when case reports and medical descriptions became much more specific. Numerous descriptions of modern day motor speech disorders can be found in medical texts from that period. For instance, in his 1817 account of his patients' "shaking palsy," James Parkinson (1755–1824) described their speech with enough detail for us to clearly recognize the characteristics of the motor speech disorder that is known today as hypokinetic dysarthria (Darley, 1983).

In 1877, Charcot described the speech of individuals with multiple sclerosis (MS), saying that, "The affected person speaks in a slow drawling manner, and sometimes almost unintelligibly. . . . The words are as if measured or scanned; there is a pause after every syllable, and syllables themselves are pronounced slowly" (Darley, 1983, p. xiv). The speech deficits described so clearly by Charcot most resemble the motor speech disorder called ataxic dysarthria. Today, it is known that individuals with MS can have ataxic dysarthria, although it is more typical for them to have another type of dysarthria, known as mixed dysarthria.

In their 1897 paper on the speech and language abilities of individuals with right hemisphere lesions, Marie and Kattwinkel described yet another type of dysarthria. They reported that the most obvious speech or language deficit after right hemisphere damage was " the mechanical functioning of speech, the articulation of words; it is really a question of *dysarthria* and not of aphasia" (Cole & Cole, 1971, p. 24). This type of dysarthria is now called unilateral upper motor neuron dysarthria and, just as described in 1897, it is primarily a disorder of articulation.

Liepmann is credited with being the first to clearly describe apraxia of speech, which, as mentioned at the beginning of this chapter, is a deficit in an individual's ability to sequence the voluntary motor movements needed to produce speech fluently (Wertz, LaPointe, & Rosenbek, 1991). Although his 1900 report was mostly a description of his patient's limb apraxia (i.e., difficulties in sequencing the movements of the limbs), Liepmann also included detailed discussions of the patient's speech deficits. At about the same time, Carl Wernicke described another type of apraxia. In his last published work (in 1906), Wernicke described the characteristics of nonverbal oral apraxia, a disorder that often co-occurs with apraxia of speech. Although he was not the first to comment on this type of apraxia, his description is remarkable for its clarity and concise detail.

For example, many such patients typically cannot protrude the tongue upon command, puff out the cheeks, show their teeth, or even open their mouth without protruding their tongue, etc. The unsuccessful attempts to carry out such actions, which before this were common everyday movements, clearly reveals the loss of ability to organize the execution of such movements (Eggert, 1977, p. 229).

For today's speech-language pathologist, the work of Darley, Aronson, and Brown (1969a, 1969b, 1975) must certainly rank as one of the most important accomplishments in the field of acquired speech and language deficits. These researchers' descriptions and classification of motor speech disorders are still very much in use. Prior to their work, the medical terms used to describe the dysarthrias varied from profession to profession. Sometimes, the name of a disorder was used as the name of the associated speech deficit. For example, the term bulbar palsy would be used as the name for weakness in the facial musculature as well as for the speech deficit caused by the weakness. A dysarthria also could be known by several terms that described the characteristics of the deficit. For instance, the dysarthria associated with damage to the cerebellum might have appeared variously as scanning speech, ataxic speech, or cerebellar speech. Through their research, publications, and presentations, Darley and his colleagues introduced a more standardized method of naming and classifying motor speech disorders. Furthermore, these researchers (1969a, 1969b) also compiled an invaluable listing of the speech errors that occur in motor speech disorders.

Today, dysarthria and apraxia of speech continue to be rich areas of research, with both medical and behavioral studies examining these disorders. Researchers throughout the world are attempting to better understand the causes of these speech deficits and develop more effective treatment methods for them. Computers and other instrumentation have opened new opportunities for research that were impossible just a few years ago. The ultimate beneficiaries of this work will be the patients who have motor speech disorders.

C H A P T E R

2

Evaluation of Motor Speech Disorders

(continued)

E. Auditory Perceptual Evaluations of the Motor Speech Mechanism
1. Phonatory-Respiratory System
2. Resonation System
3. Combined Systems
4. Stress Testing of the Motor Speech Mechanism
5. Testing for Nonverbal Oral Apraxia
6. Testing for Apraxia of Speech
7. Analysis of Connected Speech
F. Summary of the Evaluation of Motor Speech Disorders
G. Study Questions
H. Appendix 2–1: Motor Speech Examination

Most beginning clinicians find evaluating and diagnosing motor speech disorders to be a challenging task for several reasons. First, it can be difficult to distinguish among the dysarthrias, because many of the speech characteristics of one dysarthria will be present in one or more of the other dysarthrias. For example, imprecise consonants and harsh vocal quality are characteristics of every one of the dysarthrias. Second, an accurate diagnosis requires clinicians to listen very carefully to determine which of their patient's speech errors are most characteristic of a suspected motor speech disorder. This skill usually is developed with experience, which, of course, is something that beginning clinicians will not have yet acquired. Finally, a detailed knowledge of the human motor system is an invaluable asset in determining which speech errors are most important in making a correct diagnosis. It takes a concerted effort to learn about the motor system, because it is such a complex organization of nerve cells and nervous system structures. However, when a clinician understands the parts and functions of the motor system, the many symptoms of motor speech disorders are less confusing than they would be otherwise. In short, the successful evaluation of motor speech disorders requires clinicians to match what they hear in a patient's speech with what they know about the functioning of the human motor system.

For beginning clinicians, the primary challenge is to become familiar with how the speech of patients with different motor speech disorders varies from one another. Inexperienced clinicians need to learn what makes flaccid dysarthria different from spastic dysarthria and what makes ataxic dysarthria different from hypokinetic dysarthria and so forth. Fortunately, the evaluation and diagnosis of motor speech disorders can be accurate if beginning clinicians learn the characteristics of motor speech disorders, become familiar with the neuromuscular bases of these disorders, and acquire hands-on practice in clinical practicum.

There are two basic methods of evaluating motor speech disorders: instrumental and perceptual analysis. The instrumentation method uses sophisticated devices to objectively measure the components of speech production. For example, nasal and oral airflow during speech can be measured precisely by computerized instruments. Other instruments can accurately detect changes in voice onset time, atypical formant frequencies in vowels, subtle loudness variations, and many additional aspects of speech production. In contrast, the perceptual analysis method of assessment employs the ears of an examiner to detect motor speech disorders. The value of the perceptual analysis method is that the ear is the ultimate judge of whether or not there is problem with an individual's speech. If a motor speech disorder cannot be detected by ear, is there actually a disorder that needs to be treated?

For several reasons, this textbook concentrates on the perceptual analysis method of evaluating motor speech disorders. Although the importance of instrumental assessment of these disorders is without question, most practicing clinicians do not have access to such devices and must rely primarily on what their ears tell them. Furthermore, instrumental assessment is described in great detail in a number of other sources. Readers wishing to learn more about instrumentation in the assessment and treatment of motor speech disorders should examine such texts as *Dysarthria and Apraxia of Speech: Perspectives on Management* (Moore, Yorkston, & Beukelman, 1991) or *Disorders of Motor Speech: Assessment, Treatment, and Clinical Characterization* (Robin, Yorkston, & Beukelman, 1996).

GOALS OF A MOTOR SPEECH EVALUATION

In many ways, the goals of a motor speech evaluation are no different from the goals of any speech-language evaluation. Haynes and Pindzola (1998) said that a speech-language evaluation is done to understand a patient's problem and to establish the beginning level of treatment. This certainly applies to a motor speech evaluation. During a motor speech evaluation, the clinician collects relevant background information about a patient and then asks the patient to perform numerous tasks to assess the function of his or her motor speech system. Once this information is collected, the clinician should have a good description and understanding of the patient's speech abilities. With this knowledge, the clinician also has the starting place to document the effects of any treatment that may be recommended.

Duffy (1995), Swigert (1997), and other writers have suggested specific questions that clinicians should ask themselves during a motor speech evaluation. This list of questions is designed to lead clinicians to a correct diagnosis (Duffy, 1995). In fact, it is not an exaggeration to say that the primary purpose of a motor speech evaluation is to obtain the information necessary to answer these questions. If a clinician can answer each of these questions with a *detailed, informed,* and *accurate* response, the evaluation will be nearly complete.

1. Is there a problem with the patient's speech?
2. If there is a problem, what is the best way to describe it?
3. Does the problem seem to be the result of a neurologic disorder?
4. If it seems to be neurologic in origin, did it appear suddenly or slowly?
5. Is the problem related strictly to speech production or is it more of a problem with language, such as aphasia?
6. If it is a problem of speech production, do most of the problems seem to be related to the sequencing of phonemes (i.e., apraxia of speech)?
7. If there are no phoneme sequencing errors, what are the characteristics of the patient's speech errors and any associated motor problems?

The last two questions lead to the final steps in a motor speech evaluation. Question 6 is asking if the patient's speech disorder is dysarthria or apraxia of speech. Question 7 asks which type of dysarthria might be present. If clinicians are able answer these seven questions with confidence, an accurate diagnosis will be likely.

SPEECH PRODUCTION COMPONENTS AND DISORDERS

Speech does not just happen. It is dependent on the coordinated interactions of five components (or processes) that are essential for normal speech production. These components are respiration, phonation, resonance, articulation, and prosody. These five components must work together and be combined smoothly if speech is going to be produced normally. When one or any combination of the five is affected by a neuromotor disturbance, the result will be a motor speech disorder, either dysarthria or apraxia of speech.

Dysarthria is a speech production deficit that results from neuromotor damage to the peripheral or central nervous system. This damage affects any of the five components of speech production. Dysarthria is not a language disorder such as aphasia or a cognitive disorder such as dementia. Likewise, dysarthria is not a result of abnormal anatomical structure (e.g., cleft palate), sensory loss (e.g., deafness), or psychological disturbance. It is strictly a speech production disorder caused by neuromotor damage. There are actually a number of different types of dysarthria, with each having its own characteristics. Table 2–1 lists the etiologies and some of the more obvious characteristics of the various dysarthrias.

Apraxia of speech is a motor speech disorder defined as a deficit in the ability to sequence the motor commands needed to correctly position the articulators during the voluntary production of phonemes. Although it is the result of central nervous system damage, the sequencing problem in apraxia of speech is not the result of muscle weakness or slowness. As with dysarthria, apraxia of speech is not a language or cognitive disorder, or the result of anatomical, sensory, or psychological disorders. It is a disorder in the ability to sequence the motor commands needed to move the articulators smoothly from one position to another during the production of voluntary speech.

As mentioned, when any of the five components of speech production are affected by a neuromotor disorder, dysarthria or apraxia of speech will result. (Whether it is one or the other depends on where the disorder occurs in the nervous system. Apraxia of speech is nearly always associated with damage to the left hemisphere of the brain. Dysarthria, in contrast, can be caused by damage to many parts of the nervous system.)

Because the five components of speech production play such important roles in motor speech disorders, each will be discussed separately.

Respiration

Of course, the primary function of respiration is to exchange oxygen from the atmosphere for carbon dioxide from cells in the body. By

Table 2–1. The Primary Etiologies and Characteristics of the Various Dysarthrias

Type of Dysarthria	Caused By	Primary Characteristics
1. Flaccid	Damage to the cranial nerves, spinal nerves, or the neuromuscular junction.	Muscle weakness that can result in imprecise consonants, breathy phonation, hypernasality, shallow breath support, and abnormal prosody.
2. Spastic	Bilateral damage to the upper motor neurons of the pyramidal and extrapyramidal systems; often caused by brain-stem strokes.	Spasticity and weakness in the speech musculature that results in harsh or strained-strangled phonation, imprecise consonants, hypernasality, and abnormal prosody.
3. Unilateral Upper Motor Neuron	Unilateral damage to upper motor neurons.	Imprecise consonants are the most common characteristic. There may be irregular articulatory breakdowns or harsh vocal quality in some patients.
4. Ataxic	Damage to the cerebellum or the neural tracts that connect the cerebellum to the rest of the central nervous system.	Problems controlling the timing and force of speech movements, resulting in speech that often has a "drunken" quality. Imprecise consonants, distorted vowels, irregular articulatory breakdowns, and abnormal prosody.
5. Hypokinetic	A reduction of dopamine in part of the basal ganglia. Parkinsonism is the most common cause of this dysarthia.	A reduction in the range and speed of speech movements. Harsh or breathy phonation, imprecise consonants, and abnormal prosody. In some patients, there is increased rate of speech.

Table 2–1. *(continued)*

Type of Dysarthria	Caused By	Primary Characteristics
6. Hyperkinetic	Often associated with damage to the basal ganglia, but in some conditions the cause is unknown.	Involutary movements that interfere with normal speech production. Unexpected inhalations and exhalations, irregular articulatory breakdowns, and abnormal prosody.
7. Mixed	Neurological damage that extends to more than one portion of the motor system.	Any combination of the characteristics of the six pure dysarthrias. For example, a patient with parkinsonism could have a brainstem stroke that might result in a hypokinetic-spastic mixed dysarthria

exchanging these gases, respiration maintains life. Respiration also is essential for speech production. It provides the subglottic air pressure that is needed to set the vocal folds into vibration. Speech production depends on a full, steady supply of air—especially for connected speech. If the air supply is not full or steady, speech production is affected. For example, if the nerves that innervate the respiratory muscles are damaged, those muscles will be weak and may not be able to move as much air into and out of the lungs as they normally would. Therefore, nerve damage means less air for speech production, which limits the affected individual's ability to speak in anything but short phrases. In addition, respiratory deficits that reduce the amount of air available for speech can also cause reduced loudness and breathy voice quality.

Phonation

Phonation is the production of voiced phonemes through vocal fold vibrations in the larynx. Normal phonation is dependent on the complete adduction of the vocal folds and enough subglottic air pressure to set the vocal folds into vibration. The adduction of the vocal folds needs to be at just the right amount of tension to produce a clear phonation. Neuromotor damage to the nerves that innervate the vocal fold adductor muscles can have several effects on speech production. In conditions such as flaccid dysarthria, the damage may cause the adduction to be weak or incomplete. This weakness results in phonations that have a breathy or harsh quality. In conditions such as spastic dysarthria, the damage can cause the adduction to be too tight, which causes the phonation to have a strained-strangled quality. Neuromotor damage to the laryngeal muscles also may reduce the ability to change pitch or loudness during phonation.

Resonance

In motor speech disorders, resonance is the proper placement of oral or nasal tonality onto phonemes during speech. This is accomplished by the raising and lowering of the velum. Oral resonance is produced when the velum is raised and closes off the nasal cavity from the vocal airstream. This sends the sounds through the oral cavity. Nasal resonance is produced when the velum is lowered and the oral cavity is blocked by the lips or tongue, which thereby directs the entire airstream out through the nose. The key factor in this process is the movement of the velum. The muscles in the velum need to respond quickly to the different resonance requirements of the phonemes being produced during speech. When the nerves innervating these velar muscles are damaged, the muscles may be weakened or their movements slowed. Weak or slow velar muscles cannot raise the velum completely to separate the nasal cavity from the vocal airstream during the production of nonnasal speech phonemes. The resulting speech will have a hypernasal quality because nasal resonance is being applied to phonemes that ordinarily have only oral resonance.

Articulation

Articulation is the shaping of the vocal airstream into phonemes. The shaping of the airstream is accomplished in different ways. The airstream may be blocked for stop and affricate phonemes, tightly restricted for fricative phonemes, slightly restricted for semivowels, or relatively unrestricted for vowels. The shaping of the airstream happens at various points along the vocal tract. It also is accomplished by different structures within the vocal tract, known as articulators. Correct articulation requires the articulators to perform movements that have the appropriate timing, direction, force, speed, and placement for any given phoneme. By any measure, accurate articulation is the result of a very complex series of movements.

Unfortunately, neuromotor damage often affects the articulators, because most of them use muscular contractions to shape the vocal tract. When neuromotor damage affects the muscles of the lips, tongue, jaw, velum, or vocal folds, articulation is impaired. The degree of impairment depends on the severity of the damage and which articulators are affected most severely. The articulation errors that can be heard after neuromotor damage include imprecise consonants, distorted vowels, inappropriate silences, and irregular articulatory breakdowns.

Prosody

Prosody is the melody of speech. In most instances, prosody conveys meaning within an utterance through the use of stress and intonation. Stress is accomplished by changing the pitch, loudness, and duration of syllables within words to give those words added importance or to clarify meaning. Intonation is the use of pitch changes and stress to communicate, for example, whether an utterance is a question, assertion, or exclamation. Adding prosody to an utterance is not a simple task. If the prosodic features of a message are to be accurate and clear, it requires the coordinated participation of phonation, respiration, resonance, and articulation. For example, to increase the loudness of a syllable or word, there must be an increased exhalation of air from the lungs that is coordinated with a simultaneous tensing of the vocal folds. To change pitch, the vocal folds must be lengthened or shortened, which is accomplished by the simultaneous actions of several laryngeal muscles. To increase the duration of a syllable, the articulators must be held in their position for a moment longer than usual in coordination with a prolongation of phonation. The interactions of all of these vocal tract structures must be precise or prosody will sound abnormal.

Given that prosody is so dependent on the complex interaction of the other components of speech production, it should be easy to understand that neuromotor damage can affect prosody in a number of different ways. For example, if the damage causes weakness or slowness in the muscles of respiration and phonation, the strength of these muscles and the timing of their contractions will be impaired. The resulting speech may have a monopitch and monoloud quality. If the damage causes involuntary movements of the vocal tract muscles, the involuntary movements will interfere with voluntary speech movements. The resulting speech may have irregular pitch variations, sudden increases or decreases in loudness, and prolonged intervals between syllables or words.

CONDUCTING A MOTOR SPEECH EXAMINATION

The following pages of this chapter contain a complete, detailed motor speech examination form (Appendix 2–1). The tasks on this evaluation were collected and adapted from a variety of sources including the Marshfield Clinic Motor Speech Examination (unpublished), Darley et al. (1975), and Wertz et al. (1991). When conducting this motor speech examination, a clinician will be assessing the components of a patient's motor speech system.

Respiration, phonation, articulation, resonance, and prosody are all examined by the evaluation's tasks. However, a clinician also should be careful to assess more than just the five components of speech production. *As the evaluation is administered, the clinician needs to constantly assess the patient's muscle strength, speed of movement, range of motion, accuracy of movement, motor steadiness, and muscle tone.* These neuromuscular processes are the foundation of all voluntary movement in the body. Darley et al. (1975) called these six processes the "salient features" of neuromuscular function. Each of these salient features makes its own contribution to normal speech production. If any of these are defective, the motor speech system will be affected adversely. Moreover, the nature and degree of a defect can provide important information for making a correct diagnosis. That is why the features need to be examined carefully during a motor speech examination.

Muscle Strength

If a muscle within the motor speech mechanism does not have adequate strength, it may not be able to perform its speech production tasks adequately. Decreased muscle strength anywhere in the motor speech mechanism can affect respiration, articulation, resonance, phonation, and prosody. Muscle strength is assessed in numerous sections of this book's motor speech evaluation protocol. For example, a patient is asked to press his or her tongue against a tongue blade or asked to count out loud from 1 to 100 (a task known as *stress testing* the speech mechanism).

Speed of Movement

Accurate speech requires very rapid muscle movements. The tongue and vocal folds, in particular, make many rapid movements during the production of even a short utterance. Reduced speed of movement is a common characteristic of most dysarthrias. There also is one dysarthria, hypokinetic dysarthria, in which there may be increased speed of movement. Speed of movement is assessed through tasks that concentrate on alternate motion rates (AMR) and sequential motion rates (SMR). AMR tasks move the articulators through a single series of rapid back and forth movements, such as repeating "puh, puh, puh" or "tuh, tuh, tuh" as rapidly as possible. SMR tasks, in contrast, move the articulators repeatedly through a quick sequence of movements, such as repeating "puh, tuh, kuh" on one breath of air. Both AMR and SMR tasks are included in the protocol.

Range of Movement

Range of movement is how far the articulators can travel during the course of a movement. Instances of reduced range of movement include an inability to fully open the jaw or completely adduct the vocal folds. Darley et al. (1975) and Duffy (1995) both mentioned that prosody, especially, could be affected by reduced range of movement in the articulators. Range of movement is assessed most directly in the first portion of the protocol where the patient is asked to extend or hold the articulators in various positions.

Accuracy of Movement

Clear speech production requires accurate movements by the articulators. An accurate movement is one in which strength, speed, range, direction, and timing are precisely coordinated (Darley et al., 1975). If any of these are out of sync, the result can be an inaccurate movement, causing such problems as a distorted consonant or intermittent hypernasality. The AMR and SMR tasks are good for assessing the accuracy of movement, as are conversational speech and spoken paragraph reading.

Motor Steadiness

Motor steadiness is the ability to hold a body part still. There are several disorders in which involuntary movements prevent motor steadiness. The most common is tremor. These involuntary contractions can affect the laryngeal musculature and lead to a tremulous vocal quality during speech. Other disorders can cause larger, more obvious involuntary movements that interfere with all voluntary movements. In the protocol in Appendix 2–1, motor steadiness is assessed by the tasks that require a patient to hold a position or prolong a vowel. A breakdown in motor steadiness will reveal itself in an inability to maintain a still position or to produce a prolonged vowel that is smooth and steady.

Muscle Tone

Normal muscle tone is the small, constant amount of muscle contraction that is always present, even when a muscle is fully relaxed. Muscle tone maintains a muscle in a "ready to move" condition and allows for quick movement when necessary. Damage to the nervous system can alter muscle tone either by decreasing or increasing it, depending on where the damage occurs. Both circumstances can have detrimental effects on movement. Decreased muscle tone is associated with muscle weakness or paralysis. Increased tone is associated with muscle spasticity or rigidity. In the Appendix 2–1 protocol, abnormal muscle tone can be inferred by listening to the patient's speech or by looking at the affected body parts.

INSTRUCTIONS FOR THE MOTOR SPEECH EXAMINATION

Because most readers of this textbook probably have not administered many motor speech evaluations, the following pages offer a step-by-step explanation of what each task is assessing. When appropriate, an explanation of the importance of a task is provided. The entire evaluation takes between 30 and 60 minutes to administer, depending on the capabilities of the patient. Once the evaluation is completed, the clinician will have fully assessed and described the patient's speech production abilities. From the information collected about the patient, the clinician should be able to make an accurate diagnosis of a motor speech disorder that may be present.

Background Information and Medical History

This first portion of the evaluation usually is completed without too much difficulty. The information can be obtained from the patient, family members, other medical professionals, and medical records. It is important to be as thorough as possible when collecting this information, because it can provide many clues leading to a correct diagnosis. For example, a slow development of the problem may indicate a progressive neurological disorder. On the other hand, a rapid onset might suggest that an acute condition caused the disorder, perhaps a stroke. Medical records can provide important information on the patient's medical history, possible site of lesion, and current status of the problem. Rosenbek, LaPointe, and Wertz (1989) recommended that the following information be obtained from medical records:

1. The primary and secondary medical diagnoses, along with descriptions of the major symptoms
2. The date when the condition was first noted, sometimes called the "date of onset"
3. Information on the site of lesion (i. e., the place in the nervous system where the damage has occurred)
4. Earlier instances of nervous system damage
5. Evidence of limb involvement, such as weakness, involuntary movements, or motor sequencing problems (limb apraxia)
6. Information on the patient's visual acuity, including any evidence of visual field deficits
7. Information on the patient's hearing acuity

If the patient is being interviewed for this section, the clinician also can learn much about the patient's awareness and reaction to the problem. Some individuals may recognize that their speech is different, yet are not worried about it. Others may appear to be very troubled by a problem that is so mild as to be imperceptible to most listeners. Such information is valuable in making recommendations for treatment.

Face and Jaw Muscles at Rest and During Movement

The muscles of the patient's face are examined in this section of the evaluation. The clinician is looking for any abnormal muscle tone or strength, asymmetrical facial features, and restricted range of movement. The functioning of the facial cranial nerve (VII) is being assessed on most of these tasks, because it provides motor innervation to the facial muscles. The trigeminal cranial nerve (V) is examined during the tasks that require jaw movements.

Explanation of Specific Tasks

1. **Is the mouth symmetric?** Here the examiner is looking for any signs of lower face paralysis or weakness, which can cause one side of the mouth to droop lower than the other side. Be aware, however, that a small amount of mouth asymmetry is normal and does not necessarily indicate a neuromuscular disorder.

2. **Can the examiner force the lips open?** On this task the examiner is checking for muscle strength. Of course, the side of the mouth that is drooping will almost always be the weaker side. This will be the side that one should be able to force open more easily with the fingers.

3. **Does the face have an expressionless, masklike appearance?** This task checks for one of the more obvious symptoms of parkinsonism (see Chapter 8). Individuals with parkinsonism frequently have a reduced ability to express emotion through their facial expressions. Individuals with moderate and severe parkinsonism may consistently show a blank facial expression, no matter what their internal emotional state may be.

4. **When the patient looks up, is there wrinkling on both halves of the forehead?** This task assesses the possible site of neurological damage. If the damage has occurred to the facial cranial nerve (VII) near where it branches out from the brainstem, the entire half of the affected side of the face will be weakened or paralyzed. In this situation, there will be no wrinkling of the skin of the forehead when the patient looks up, because the forehead muscles will not contract normally. If, however, the damage has occurred to either the left or right tract of the upper motor neurons, there will most likely be movement in the muscles on both sides of the forehead, with only the lower face showing evidence of weakness or paralysis. This is because the upper branch of the facial cranial nerve that serves the forehead muscles receives *bilateral* innervation from the upper motor neurons, but the lower branch serving the lower face receives only *unilateral* innervation from the upper motor neurons. The innervation of the facial muscles is explained in more detail in Chapter 4.

5. **Is the patient's smile symmetric?** This task, as well as the next two, looks at voluntary movement of the lower face muscles. The examiner is checking for any evidence of weakness or reduced range of motion. In addition, the clinician needs to check for signs of the patient appearing to grope for the correct position to accomplish this task. If groping is present, it may be evidence of a nonverbal oral apraxia. In such a case, be sure to administer the portions of the protocol covering apraxia. Apraxia is covered in Chapter 11.

6. **Is the patient able to pucker his or her lips?** This task assesses muscular strength and range of movement of the orbicularis oris muscles of the lips. Weakness on one side of the mouth may result in an asymmetrical puckering of the lips.

7. **Is the patient able to puff out his or her cheeks and hold the air in the oral cavity as you squeeze the cheeks?** Here the examiner is assessing the strength of the lips and the velum to maintain an airtight seal. Weakness at either end will result in leakage of air out of the mouth or the nose when pressure is applied to the patient's cheeks. Look closely at the lips as the cheeks are squeezed to determine if that is where air is escaping. If you are confident that the lip seal is tight, any leakage is probably occurring at the velopharyngeal port. The function of the velum is assessed on several additional tasks later in the protocol.

8. **Does the jaw hang loosely?** If so, this would suggest significant bilateral damage to the trigeminal cranial nerve (V), which innervates the jaw muscles. However, bilateral damage is not common. Typically, damage affects only one side. When the damage is only on one side of the jaw, the muscles on the unaffected side will provide more than enough strength to hold the jaw in a normal position.

9. **Does the jaw deviate to one side when the mouth is wide open?** This task checks for unilateral damage to the trigeminal cranial nerve. When the jaw muscles on one side of the face are weaker than on the other side, the jaw may deviate to the weaker side when the mouth is opened widely.

10. **Is the patient able to move the jaw from to the right and left?** An inability to do this suggests bilateral weakness of the jaw muscles. However, hesitations or groping on this task also might indicate a nonverbal oral apraxia.

11. **Is the patient able to keep the jaw closed while the examiner attempts to open it?** This task assesses the strength of the muscles that elevate the jaw, primarily the masseter and

temporalis. If you are able to manually open the jaw, it suggests bilateral weakness in these muscles—possibly the result of bilateral damage to the trigeminal cranial nerve.

12. **Is the patient able to keep the jaw open while the examiner attempts to close it?** This task examines the muscles that open the jaw. These muscles are the digastricus, mylohyoid, and geniohyoid. If you can manually close the jaw while the patient attempts to keep it open, bilateral weakness of these muscles is indicated.

Tongue at Rest and During Movement

Of course, the tongue is one of the key articulators. Impairments to its structure or function can have significant effects on the articulation of speech sounds. It is especially important to evaluate the tongue at rest and during movement. Both positions can provide important diagnostic information. Most of the assessment tasks in this section examine the function of the hypoglossal cranial nerve (XII), which innervates the intrinsic and extrinsic muscles of the tongue. If groping tongue movements are noted in any of these tasks, be sure to complete the apraxia section of the evaluation.

Explanation of Specific Tasks

1. **Does the size of the tongue appear normal at rest?** When damage occurs to lower motor neurons (such as those in the cranial nerves), the muscles normally innervated by those neurons will shrink because of atrophy. If there is unilateral damage to the hypoglossal nerve, the half of the tongue that is on the same side as the damage can take on a furrowed, shrunken appearance. When this damage occurs to both the left and right hypoglossal cranial nerves, the muscle atrophy will affect the whole tongue, leaving the entire tongue shrunken.

2. **Is the tongue symmetric at rest?** If damage to the hypoglossal cranial nerve (XII) is restricted to only one side, the resulting atrophy will be restricted to that same side. The tongue will consequently have an asymmetrical appearance, with the unaffected side looking normal and only the other side demonstrating the atrophy.

3. **Are fasciculations present when the tongue is at rest?** Fasciculations are small involuntary movements that may

occur in a muscle when motor innervation has been lost through damage to lower motor neurons. If fasciculations are present after damage to the hypoglossal cranial nerve, you will see small, nonrhythmic dimpling along the surface of the tongue, or you might see subtle "wormlike" movements of the entire tongue.

4. **Does the tongue remain still while at rest?** In addition to fasciculations, other conditions can result in involuntary movements when the tongue is supposedly at rest. Such hyperkinetic movement disorders as chorea and dystonia may cause the tongue to involuntarily protrude, retract, rotate, and move side-to-side. Hyperkinetic movement disorders are discussed in Chapter 9.

5. **Is the patient able to protrude the tongue completely?** This assesses range of motion for the posterior fibers of the genioglossus muscle, which protrudes the tongue, and the vertical and transverse intrinsic muscles, which give the tongue its "pointed" shape when protruded. If there is bilateral weakness of these muscles, the tongue can only be protruded a limited distance, if at all. If the weakness is unilateral, the protruded tongue will deviate to the affected side. This deviation to the affected side is the result of unequal contractions of the left and right sides of the genioglosssus muscle in the tongue. The contractions of the unaffected side of this muscle will overcome the weakened contractions on the other side of the muscle, thereby causing the tongue to point to the affected side. You can check the strength of tongue protrusion by having the patient push the tongue against a tongue blade held firmly in front of the mouth.

6. **Can the patient keep the tongue tip at midline while the examiner pushes the tongue to the left and right?** This task checks the strength of several tongue muscles, including the genioglossus, superior longitudinal, and inferior longitudinal muscles.

7. **Is the patient able to touch the upper lip with the tongue tip?** Here you are assessing the range of motion of the tongue protrusion muscles (genioglossus, vertical and transverse intrinsic muscles) and the superior longitudinal muscle, which elevates the tongue tip.

8. **Can the patient keep the tongue tip pressed against the inside of the cheek as the examiner pushes the cheek inward?** This is an examination of strength for a number of tongue muscles, primarily the longitudinal muscles. The tongue tip will

deviate to the left or right with simultaneous contraction of either the left or right superior and inferior longitudinal muscles, respectively. Unilateral weakness in these muscles is evident through comparison of the amount of outward force the tongue is able to apply to either the right or left cheek.

9. **Can the patient move the tongue from side-to-side?** This task examines range of motion for the superior and inferior longitudinal muscles. These muscles are used to lateralize the tongue from one corner of the mouth to the other. Reduced lateral tongue movement to one side of the mouth will reveal unilateral weakness of these muscles.

Velum and Pharynx at Rest and During Movement

This section of the evaluation looks at the structure and function of the velum and pharynx. Most of the muscles in these structures are innervated by the vagus cranial nerve (X). It is difficult to obtain much in-depth information about these structures in this portion of the examination because they are difficult to see clearly. In truth, you are only able to look for the most obvious anatomical and functional deviations. Additional information about the velum and pharynx can be obtained in later sections of this examination.

Explanation of Specific Tasks

1. **Does the velum rise symmetrically each time the patient says /a/?** Have the patient repeat /a/ 4 or 5 times. Make sure there is a brief pause between each production. This will allow the velum to return to its resting position after each /a/, giving one a better opportunity to observe the full range of velar movement. A normally functioning velum and pharynx work together to close the velopharyngeal port during the production of nonnasal sounds. You should see the entire velum rise promptly just before phonation. At the same time, the sides and back of the upper pharynx should move slightly inward to meet the rising velum.

In cases of moderate to severe bilateral weakness of the velum and pharynx, you should be able to observe reduced speed and range of motion of these structures when the patient repeats /a/. However, these reductions may be difficult to detect visually when there is mild bilateral weakness. When there is unilateral muscular weakness of the velum and pharynx, the unaffected side should demonstrate nearly normal movement. The impaired side will show little or no movement. The uvula will be pulled toward the stronger, unaffected side as that side of the velum rises.

2. **Is there a pharyngeal gag reflex when the back wall of the pharynx is touched?** The gag is a protective reflex. Its purpose is to clear the upper pharynx of an obstruction that might threaten to block the airway. Testing this reflex assesses the neuromuscular loop that starts with the sensory nerves in pharyngeal muscles and tissue. When the sensory nerves in the pharynx are stimulated by the touch of a foreign object, they send a sensory impulse through the glossopharyngeal cranial nerve (IX) to the brainstem. From the brainstem, a motor impulse is sent directly out to the pharyngeal and velar muscles via the vagus cranial nerve (X), which causes those muscles to rapidly contract. Damage at any portion of this loop leads to a decreased or absent gag reflex. Note, however, that many individuals without neurological damage are quite insensitive to pharyngeal stimulation and do not readily demonstrate a gag reflex.

Laryngeal Function

The function of the larynx cannot be observed directly. To actually observe the actions of the larynx, you need instrumentation, such as a laryngeal mirror or a flexible nasoendoscope. However, there are procedures to indirectly assess laryngeal function. The following three tasks evaluate the strength and range of movement of the laryngeal adductor and abductor muscles. Other tasks later in the evaluation assess phonation, which is a key function of the larynx.

Explanations of Specific Tasks

1. **Is the patient able to produce a sharp cough?** This task assesses the strength of vocal fold adduction. Producing a sharp cough requires tight vocal fold adduction for building up subglottic air pressure. In cases in which adduction is weak, the cough will have a soft, breathy quality because the

adductor muscles are not strong enough to hold air in the lungs. In some instances, this task also assesses the adequacy of the respiratory system. If the respiratory muscles are not strong enough to provide a forced exhalation of air, the resulting cough also will have that soft, breathy quality. The next step of this evaluation presents a procedure for determining whether a breathy cough is the result of laryngeal or respiratory weakness.

2. **Can the patient produce a sharp glottal stop?** In this task the patient is asked to produce an abrupt glottal stop (or a forceful grunt) to assess the strength of vocal fold adduction. Duffy (1995) recommended this procedure to help determine if a weak cough is the result of inadequate vocal fold adduction or poor breath support. If a patient who produces a weak cough can bring the vocal folds together with enough force to make a sharp glottal stop, then he or she has sufficient adductor muscle strength to close the glottis tightly. This would suggest that a weak cough is the result of poor breath support, not adductor muscle weakness.

3. **Is inhalatory stridor present?** If abductor muscle paralysis prevents the vocal folds from being abducted completely, a patient may demonstrate inhalatory stridor, which is a breathy wheeze that can be heard during inhalation. This vocal fold abductor paralysis may be caused by unilateral or bilateral damage to the vagus cranial nerve. In severe cases, the stridor is actually a phonation on inhalation. Although stridor may be evident on quiet breathing, you will probably need to ask most patients to take a quick, deep breath before it will be noticeable.

AUDITORY-PERCEPTUAL EVALUATIONS OF THE MOTOR SPEECH MECHANISM

In most cases, the ear is the best instrument for evaluating deficits of the motor speech mechanism. A clinician with an experienced ear can often make a quick, accurate diagnosis based only on the acoustic characteristics of a patient's speech. The importance of developing a sharp ear for the assessment of motor speech disorders cannot be overstated. After all, what a listener hears with his or her ears provides the ultimate judgment of whether speech production is defective. Accordingly, most of the remaining evaluation tasks rely on a clinician's perceptual analysis of a patient's speech.

Phonatory-Respiratory System

It is logical to assess the phonatory and repiratory components of the speech mechanism at the same time, because normal phonation is so dependent on an adequate supply of subglottic air pressure. In this protocol section, the clinician will determine the length of time the patient can prolong an /a/. One should listen critically to the quality, pitch, and loudness of the patient's phonation, because each of these characteristics can provide much useful diagnostic information.

Explanations of Specific Tasks

1. **"Take a deep breath and say /a/ as long, steadily, and clearly as you can."** This task assesses both the adequacy of breath support and vocal fold adduction for phonation. If there is too little breath support, there will be inadequate subglottic air pressure to prolong the /a/ for 15 seconds. If the vocal folds are not adducted fully, excess amounts of air will escape from the larynx during phonation. This wastes subglottic air and lessens the length of the phonation. To determine if a reduced length of phonation is the result of poor breath support or incomplete vocal fold adduction, check the results from the previous section of the evaluation, which provided for assessment of the adequacy of vocal fold adduction.

2. **Is there a latency period between the signal to say /a/ and the initiation of phonation?** If there is a delay, it may be the result of weakness in the phonatory-respiratory system. It also could be the result of a problem of sequencing the motor movements needed to produce the /a/. Such sequencing difficulties are characteristic of apraxia, which is assessed in greater detail later in the evaluation.

3. **Quality, Pitch, and Loudness of Phonations.** In a normal phonation, the vocal quality is steady, even, smooth, and clear. The presence of **hypernasality** indicates inadequate velopharyngeal closure. **Breathiness** can indicate incomplete vocal fold adduction during phonation. **Harshness** is an abnormal vocal quality that is caused by the friction of air being passed through vocal folds that are *almost* adducted fully. **Diplophonia** is the simultaneous production of two pitch levels during phonation. In motor speech disorders, it is usually the result of unilateral vocal fold paralysis.

Pitch can be affected by motor speech disorders. It may be **too low**, as in spastic dysarthria and several of the hyperkinetic dysarthrias. There may be a **tremor** in the phonations, which usually is present in essential voice tremor, one of the hyperkinetic dysarthrias. **Pitch breaks** are sudden shifts in pitch during phonation. These are heard most often in flaccid and spastic dysarthria.

Loudness can be affected by motor speech disorders. The involuntary movements in hyperkinetic dysarthria can cause **excessive loudness variations** during phonations. Poor respiratory support or inadequate phonation can cause **decreased loudness**, perhaps most often heard in flaccid and hypokinetic dysarthria.

Resonation System

This portion of the evaluation assesses velopharyngeal function. Weakened or paralyzed velar muscles result in incomplete velopharyngeal closure, which is heard perceptually as hypernasality. In motor speech disorders, hypernasality is most frequently a symptom of flaccid, spastic, and hypokinetic dysarthria. Hyponasality, the counterpart of hypernasality, is rarely present in the speech of individuals with dysarthria or apraxia of speech. Because other tasks in this motor speech evaluation have already evaluated elements of the resonatory system (velar movement, hypernasal voice quality), the findings of the following two tasks should be combined with the results of the previous tasks to arrive at the most accurate assessment of the patient's velopharyngeal function.

Explanations of Specific Tasks

1. **"Take a deep breath and say /u/ for as long as you can."** On this task, the clinician asks the patient to prolong the high, back vowel /u/, which usually maximizes velopharyngeal closure. While the patient says /u/, the clinician holds a small mirror first under one nostril and then under the other. Nasal emission of air during this phonation will be revealed as fogging of the mirror. You should disregard any momentary fogging of the mirror at the very beginning or end of the phonation. However, the mirror should remain clear during the middle of the phonation.

2. "This time I'm going to squeeze your nose. Don't let it bother you." Here the clinician makes a perceptual judgment of whether hypernasality is present during the prolongation of /u/. By alternately squeezing and releasing the nostrils while the patient is producing /u/, you are intermittently stopping any nasal airflow during phonation. If there is hypernasality, you will hear a difference in resonance as the patient's nose is squeezed and released.

Combined Systems (Phonation, Respiration, Resonance, and Articulation)

Alternate motion rate (AMR) is an assessment of a patient's ability to move the articulators rapidly yet smoothly in a repetitive motion. It also is known sometimes as the diadochokinetic rate. AMRs are a key evaluation task for motor speech disorders. They provide valuable information on the speed and rhythm of syllable production. AMRs are very important in a motor speech evaluation, because individuals with different types of dysarthria typically perform differently on this task:

- Individuals with flaccid and spastic dysarthria usually have slow and regular AMRs.
- Individuals with ataxic and hyperkinetic dysarthria often have slow and irregular AMRs.
- Some individuals with hypokinetic dysarthria have AMRs that are more rapid than normal. In certain individuals with this dysarthria, the AMRs are said so quickly that their articulation of the phonemes is blurred.

By carefully analyzing the patient's AMR performance, one can often obtain important diagnostic information about the patient's dysarthria.

Explanation of Specific Task

"Take a deep breath and say "puh, puh, puh" as long, as fast, and as evenly as you can." After saying these directions, be sure to demonstrate for the patient how the syllables should be produced. To obtain an accurate count of the patient's AMRs, it is important to always use some type of instrumentation during this task, either a Visi-Pitch, a tape recorder, or some other recording device. Even experienced clinicians have difficulty

timing and counting syllable repetitions, if the patient's performance is not recorded. In this task, you are primarily listening
for the speed and rhythm of the productions, but loudness, pitch,
and articulation also are important. For example, excessive variations in syllable loudness are typical of ataxic and hyperkinetic
dysarthria; blurred articulation can be a characteristic of hypokinetic dysarthria.

Sequential motion rate (SMR) is a task that assesses a patient's
ability to move the articulators in a rapid, smooth sequence of
motions. Typically, SMRs are more difficult to perform accurately
than AMRs. This task is especially useful in bringing out the symptoms of apraxia of speech. It is not unusual to have individuals
with apraxia of speech complete the AMR task successfully but be
unable to complete even the first attempt at the SMR sequence.
Some of the errors individuals with apraxia of speech may demonstrate on the SMR task include delays in beginning the task,
phoneme substitutions, incorrect sequencing of syllables, and articulatory groping for the correct phoneme placement. This is not to
suggest, however, that all individuals with apraxia of speech are
able to complete the AMR task successfully. Many have difficulty
with both tasks.

Explanation of Specific Task

"Now I want you to make those three sounds together." As
with the AMRs, it is important to record the patient's trials on
the SMR task to obtain an accurate syllable count. One should
also be sure to demonstrate for the patient how the syllables
should be produced.

Stress Testing of the Motor Speech Mechanism

This task is a screening for myasthenia gravis, a disorder that causes a
rapid fatigue of the muscles during a sustained motor activity (see
Chapter 4). To test for myasthenia gravis, ask the patient to count
quickly from 1 to 100. Listen for a relatively rapid deterioration of
articulation, resonance, or phonation while the patient is counting.
Typically, there will be a recovery of muscle function after a rest period, but performance will decline if the muscles again are taxed in a
sustained activity.

Testing for Nonverbal Oral Apraxia

Apraxia is a disruption in the ability to voluntarily sequence complex movements accurately. It is not the result of muscle weakness, reduced range of motion, or a cognitive inability to plan the target movement. Apraxia is a problem in sequencing the steps of a complex movement that has already been planned by the higher centers of the brain. There are two types of apraxia that can affect the speech musculature: nonverbal oral apraxia and apraxia of speech. Nonverbal oral apraxia is a disruption in the sequencing of oral movements that are nonverbal, sometimes described as vegetative movements. Examples of nonverbal oral movements include smiling, puckering the lips, protruding the tongue, and biting the lower lip. Individuals with this type of apraxia will demonstrate hesitations, groping, and revisions when attempting to perform nonverbal oral movements. It is possible for someone to have nonverbal oral apraxia but not have apraxia of speech. It is also possible for someone to have apraxia of speech but not nonverbal oral apraxia. Usually, however, these two types of apraxia are cooccurring disorders, which means that if one is present, so is the other.

Explanation of Specific Task

> **"Now I want you to do some things."** These tasks assess the patient's ability to perform voluntary nonverbal oral movements. Do not demonstrate the desired movement for the patient immediately after reading the command. Wait until the patient has attempted the task independently before demonstrating the movement. The patient's performance is graded on an 11-point scale, which ranges from a prompt response to no oral movement. Such a scoring system allows the clinician to obtain a much more detailed picture of a patient's performance than a simple right or wrong scoring. One should become familiar with the 11 points before administering this portion of the evaluation.

Testing for Apraxia of Speech

Apraxia of speech is the other type of apraxia that can affect the speech musculature. It is a disruption in the sequencing of voluntary movements for speech production. Individuals with apraxia of speech often demonstrate numerous sequencing errors when they are attempting to speak, especially when trying to say multisyllabic words. These errors include groping to position the articulators correctly, transpositions of syllables within a word, and phoneme substitutions. Interestingly, both automatic and emotional speech are usually free of apraxic errors, which means that such verbal tasks as counting, uttering an expletive, or replying to a social greeting are often produced correctly. Apraxia of speech is discussed in more detail in Chapter 11.

Explanation of Specific Tasks

1. **"Say these words for me."** This task has the patient repeating or reading a list of words. The list starts with a two-syllable word and progresses to a complex sequence of increasingly longer words that all start with the same CVC syllable. It should be extremely difficult for an individual with apraxia of speech to complete this list without demonstrating numerous sequencing errors. Not only are most of the words multisyllabic, most of them also are low frequency words, which means that they are words that do not occur frequently in everyday conversations. Apraxic speakers usually have more difficulty pronouncing low frequency words than high frequency words.

2. **"Now these."** Individuals with apraxia of speech typically have little difficulty producing single-syllable words with a simple CVC construction in which the initial and final consonants are identical. Words of this type are included in the evaluation for two reasons. First, the patient should find them to be a successful change of pace from the difficult previous task. Second, the words provide a strong indication of severity if the patient demonstrates many apraxic errors on these words. Because they should be fairly easy for most individuals with apraxia of speech, a patient who has difficulty with these words is probably severely affected by the apraxia.

3. **"Now repeat these sentences after me."** The sentences on this task should be difficult for individuals with apraxia of speech. These items are uncommon sentences that contain numerous multisyllabic words. They should evoke some apraxic errors in most individuals suspected of having apraxia of speech.

4. **"Count from 1 to 20."** Because this is an overlearned, automatic verbal task, many individuals with apraxia of speech should be able to complete it with far fewer errors than they will demonstrate on the next task.

5. **"Now count backward from 20 to 1."** Most individuals with apraxia of speech should make multiple errors on this task, if they can complete it at all. Although they are producing the same words as in prior task, counting backwards is not an overlearned verbal activity. Consequently, this should be a difficult task for most patients with apraxia of speech.

6. **"Tell me what is happening in this picture."** This task is divided into two parts. In the first portion, the patient is asked to describe the Cookie Theft picture from the *Boston Diagnostic Examination for Aphasia*. The clinician writes down four of the sentences spoken by the patient during the description of the picture. (If the picture description does not provide four sentences, write down any sentences spoken by the patient during the evaluation.) In the second portion of this task, the patient is asked to repeat the four sentences written during the picture description.

   The rationale for this task is that fewer apraxic errors are typically noted in spontaneous utterances compared to purposeful utterances. When describing the picture, the patient is engaging in a much more spontaneous speech act than when being asked to repeat sentences. Consequently, one should expect to hear fewer errors during the picture description task than when the patient repeats his or her own utterances just minutes after first producing them.

Analysis of Connected Speech

In this final portion of the evaluation, the clinician should have the patient read one of the standard reading passages such as the Grandfather passage or the Rainbow passage. To ensure an accurate analysis of the patient's connected speech, it is very important to obtain a good quality audio or video recording of this task. Rate the characteristics of the patient's speech according to the questions listed at the end of the examination (Darley et al., 1975). A complete analysis of connected speech should provide much of the information needed to distinguish one dysarthria from another.

SUMMARY OF THE EVALUATION OF MOTOR SPEECH DISORDERS

- Evaluating motor speech disorders can be a challenging task for inexperienced clinicians. There are numerous elements of speech production that must be assessed if a proper diagnosis is to be made. The clinician needs to evaluate a patient's respiration, phonation, resonance, articulation, and prosody during a motor speech examination.
- Instrumentation and perceptual analysis are the two primary methods of assessing motor speech disorders. Most clinicians use perceptual analysis to make their diagnosis. With this method, clinicians use their eyes and ears to determine if a motor speech disorder is present in a given patient.
- In addition to evaluating the elements of speech production (e.g., respiration, phonation, and so forth), a complete motor speech examination will examine the six processes that are the foundation of all voluntary movements: muscle strength, speed of movement, range of movement, accuracy of movement, motor steadiness, and muscle tone.
- At the most basic level, a motor speech examination allows a clinician to fully describe a patient's speech production abilities. With this complete description of the patient's abilities, the clinician should be able to logically answer pertinent questions about the patient's deficits and arrive at a correct diagnosis.

STUDY QUESTIONS

1. What are the two basic methods of evaluating motor speech disorders?
2. According to Haynes and Pindzola, what are the two goals of any speech-language evaluation?
3. What are the five components of speech production?
4. Define dysarthria.
5. Define apraxia of speech.
6. What are Darley, Aronson, and Brown's salient features of neuromuscular function, and why are they important?
7. Name two evaluation tasks that assess tongue strength.
8. What are AMRs and SMRs, and why are they important?
9. What might inhalation stridor indicate?
10. Why might an individual with apraxia of speech have difficulty counting backwards from 20 to 1?

APPENDIX 2–1

Motor Speech Examination

Patient's Name:

Date of Examination:

Patient's Age:

Neurologic Diagnosis:

Relevant Personal Information:

Medical History:

Instructions: Answer each item yes or no and indicate the degree of impairment as follows:

> 0 = no impairment
> 1 = mild impairment
> 2 = moderate impairment
> 3 = severe impairment

Also be sure to answer all other questions in the space indicated.

I. STRUCTURAL-FUNCTIONAL SPEECH MECHANISM EXAMINATION

	Yes	No	Degree
A. Facial Musculature at Rest: CN VII			
1. Is mouth symmetrical?	☐	☐	_____
If no, describe: _____			
_____			
2. Can patient resist examiner's attempt to force lips open?	☐	☐	_____
3. Are eyes open?	☐	☐	_____
4. Are eyes partially closed?	☐	☐	_____
5. Is facies rigid or masked?	☐	☐	_____
6. Is there wrinkling of forehead (when looking up without moving head?)	☐	☐	_____
7. Is nose symmetrical?	☐	☐	_____
If no, describe: _____			
_____			
B. Facial Musculature During Voluntary Movement: CN VII			
1. Is smile symmetrical?	☐	☐	_____
If no, describe: _____			
_____			
2. [†]Is groping present?	☐	☐	_____
3. Can patient pucker the lips?	☐	☐	_____
If no, describe: _____			
_____			
4. [†]Is groping present?	☐	☐	_____
5. Can patient puff out cheeks and maintain lip seal when pressure is applied?	☐	☐	_____
If no, describe: _____			
_____			
C. Mandibular Musculature at Rest: CN V			
Does mandible hang lower than normal?	☐	☐	_____
D. Mandibular Musculature During Voluntary Movement: CN V			
1. When mouth is open as widely as possible, is there deviation to one side?	☐	☐	_____
If no, describe: _____			
_____			

[†]Any groping should be followed up with the complete apraxia battery.

	Yes	No	Degree
2. †Is groping present?	☐	☐	_____
3. Can patient move mandible voluntarily to the right or left?	☐	☐	_____
4. Can patient resist examiner's attempt to open lower jaw when teeth are clenched?	☐	☐	_____
5. Can patient keep mouth wide open as examiner attempts to force it closed?	☐	☐	_____

E. Tongue Musculature at Rest: CN XII

	Yes	No	Degree
1. Is tongue normal in size? If no, describe: _____	☐	☐	_____
2. Does tongue lie midline? If no, describe: _____	☐	☐	_____
3. Is the tongue symmetrical in shape? If no, describe: _____	☐	☐	_____
4. With tongue resting atop edges of lower incisor teeth, is fasciculation observable?	☐	☐	_____
5. Does tongue remain at rest? If no, describe: _____	☐	☐	_____

F. Tongue Musculature during Voluntary Movement: CN XII

	Yes	No	Degree
1. Can patient protrude tongue completely? If no, describe range and deviation: _____	☐	☐	_____
2. †Is groping present?	☐	☐	_____
3. With tongue protruded, can patient resist examiner's attempt to force tongue to other side?	☐	☐	_____
4. With tip of tongue, can patient resist examiner's attempt to force tongue to one side or other?	☐	☐	_____

†Any groping should be followed up with the complete apraxia battery.

	Yes	No	Degree
5. With tip of tongue, can patient touch: upper lip?	☐	☐	_____
alveolar ridge?	☐	☐	_____
If no, describe: _____			
6. With tongue in cheek, can patient resist examiner's effort to force tongue inward?	☐	☐	_____
7. Can the patient move the tongue from side-to-side?	☐	☐	_____
If no, describe: _____			

G. The Velum and Pharynx at Rest and During Movement: CN X
  1. Does the velum rise symmetrically each time the patient says /a/?   ☐ ☐ _____
     If no, describe: _____

  2. Is there a gag reflex when the back wall of the pharynx is touched?   ☐ ☐ _____

H. The Function of the Larynx: CN X
  1. Is the patient able to produce a sharp cough?   ☐ ☐ _____
  2. Can the patient produce a sharp glottal stop?   ☐ ☐ _____
     If no, describe: _____

  3. Is inhalatory stridor present?   ☐ ☐ _____
     If yes, describe: _____

II. ACOUSTIC MOTOR SPEECH EXAMINATION

A. Phonatory-Respiratory System:

  1. <u>Directions to patient</u>: "Take a deep breath and say /a:/ as long, steadily, and clearly as you can."

    a. Duration: Trial 1: _____

                    Trial 2: _____

                    Trial 3: _____

                    Average: _____

                    (average is 15 s for adults & 10 s for school-aged children)

	Yes	No	Degree
b. Latency: Is there a latency period between signal to say /a:./ and initiation of phonation?	☐	☐	_____
c. Quality:			
Steady and even	☐	☐	_____
Smooth and clear	☐	☐	_____
Hypernasality	☐	☐	_____
Breathiness	☐	☐	_____
Harshness	☐	☐	_____
Diplophonia	☐	☐	_____
d. Pitch			
Too high	☐	☐	_____
Too low	☐	☐	_____
Normal	☐	☐	_____
Tremor	☐	☐	_____
Pitch breaks	☐	☐	_____
e. Loudness			
Excessive loudness	☐	☐	_____
Inadequate loudness	☐	☐	_____
Normal loudness	☐	☐	_____

    f. Describe Abnormalities: _____

_____

_____

	Yes	No	Degree

B. Resonatory System:

   1. <u>Directions to patients:</u> "Take a deep breath and say /u:/ for as long as you can." Hold a (laryngeal) mirror beneath one nostril and then the other. Leakage from (L. R. Both) nostrils. ☐ ☐ _____

   2. <u>Directions to patient</u>: "Now I want you to do the same thing, but this time I'm going to squeeze your nose. Don't let it bother you; just keep the /u:/ going."

      Change in resonance when occluding (L. R. Both) nostrils. ☐ ☐ _____

      Connected speech without nasal. ☐ ☐ _____

C. Combined Systems (Phonatory, Respiratory, Resonatory, and Articulatory)

   1. *Alternate Motion Rate* (diadochokinetic) <u>Directions to patient:</u> "Take a deep breath and say (e.g., /pʌpʌpʌ/) as long, and as fast, and as evenly as you can." Demonstrate.

      Is AMR slow? ☐ ☐ _____

      Is AMR excessively fast? ☐ ☐ _____

      Is AMR dysrhythmic? ☐ ☐ _____

      Is AMR uneven in loudness? ☐ ☐ _____

      Is AMR uneven in pitch? ☐ ☐ _____

      Is there a tremor? ☐ ☐ _____

      Is there equal spacing between syllables? ☐ ☐ _____

      Is there blurring (lack of differentiation between syllables)? ☐ ☐ _____

      Is there hypernasality? ☐ ☐ _____

      Is there nasal emission? ☐ ☐ _____

      Is there restriction in amplitude of motion of lips and jaw? ☐ ☐ _____

      Are there imprecise or distorted consonants? ☐ ☐ _____

Indicate rate per 5-second interval on this table:

	/pʌ/	/tʌ/	/kʌ/	/pʌtʌkʌ/
Trial 1				
Trial 2				
Trial 3				
Average				

Average rate for /pʌ/ and /tʌ/ is about 30–35 repetitions for 5 seconds; /kʌ/ is somewhat slower.

2. Sequential *Motion Rate*

Directions to patient: "Now I want you to make those three sounds, 'puh,' 'tuh,' and 'kuh' together." Demonstrate. Note: Record the results (per 5-second trial) on the table above.

	Yes	No	Degree
a. Is patient able to move smoothly from syllable to syllable?	☐	☐	_____
b. Are sounds blocked, transposed or omitted?	☐	☐	_____

If yes, describe: _____
_____

3. Stress Testing of the Motor Speech Mechanism (screening for myasthenia gravis)

Instruct the patient to count rapidly (approximately two numbers per second) at least up through 100. Demonstrate 1–10.

Is there audible deterioration of phonation or articulation? ☐ ☐ _____

If yes, describe: _____
_____

III. TESTING FOR NONVERBAL ORAL APRAXIA

A. Tests for Nonverbal Oral Apraxia

Directions to patient: "Now I want you to do some things. Listen closely and do everything as completely and as well as you can. Are you ready?"

Response	Test Item	Graded Response Scale
_____	1. Stick out your tongue.	1. Accurate and immediate response with no hesitation.
_____	2. Show me how you blow out a match.	
_____	3. Show me your teeth.	
_____	4. Round your lips.	2. Accurate after trial-and-error searching movement on command.
_____	5. Touch your nose with the tip of your tongue.	
_____	6. Bite your lower lip.	
_____	7. Show me how you whistle.	3. Crude, defective in amplitude, accuracy, or speed on command.
_____	8. Lick your lips all around.	
_____	9. Clear your throat.	
_____	10. Move your tongue in and out.	
_____	11. Click your teeth together once.	4. Partial response (an important part missing) on command.
_____	12. Show me how you smile.	
_____	13. Click your tongue.	
_____	14. Chatter your teeth as if cold.	5. Same as (1) after demonstration.
_____	15. Touch your chin with the tip of your tongue.	6. Same as (2) after demonstration.
_____	16. Show me how you cough.	7. Same as (3) after demonstration.
_____	17. Puff out your cheeks.	
_____	18. Wiggle your tongue from side to side.	8. Same as (4) after demonstration.
_____	19. Pucker your lips.	9. Perseverative response.
_____	20. Alternately pucker and smile.	10. Irrelevant response.
		11. No oral performance.

IV. TESTING FOR APRAXIA OF SPEECH
(ORAL VERBAL APRAXIA)

Directions to patient: "Say those words for me." If patient is unable to repeat to verbal stimuli, present words as printed on cards. As patient reads or repeats the following, tape record and transcribe errors.

1. slowpoke _____
2. conference _____
3. Tahiti _____
4. dressmaker _____
5. Annapolis _____
6. kindergarten _____
7. condominium _____
8. industrial revolution _____
9. Winnie-the-Pooh and Tigger too _____
10. stiff - stiffer - stiffening _____
11. base - baseball - baseball cap _____
12. fan - fancy - fantastic - fashionable _____
13. glow - glowing - glistening - glamorously _____
14. rid - riddle - ridicule - ridiculous _____

"Now these."

mime _____   shush _____
George _____   dude _____
pipe _____   tent _____
babe _____   Nan _____

"Please repeat these sentences for me."

1. The beautiful girl was dancing. _____
_____

2. Open this birthday present first. _____
_____

3. The stranger walked into the store. _____
_____

4. The birdwatcher saw a Norwegian Blue parrot. _____
_____

"Count from 1 to 20." *Note:* Indicate pauses for breath by a slash (/) after the appropriate number.

1. _____   2. _____   3. _____   4. _____

5. _____   6. _____   7. _____   8. _____

9. _____   10. _____   11. _____   12. _____

13. _____   14. _____   15. _____   16. _____

17. _____   18. _____   19. _____   20. _____

"Now count backward from 20 to 1."

20. _____   19. _____   18. _____   17. _____

16. _____   15. _____   14. _____   13. _____

12. _____   11. _____   10. _____   9. _____

8. _____   7. _____   6. _____   5. _____

4. _____   3. _____   2. _____   1. _____

"Tell me what is happening in this picture." Use the Boston's "Cookie Theft." Evoke at least 1 minute of ongoing speech. If necessary point out neglected features of the picture by asking, "What's happening here?"

Write down any four sentences that the patient says. If the patient provides an insufficient speech sample here, use any (four) sentences produced at any point in the evaluation.

1. _____

2. _____

3. _____

4. _____

"Say these sentences after me." Use any (four) sentences just written above. Write down (and if necessary, phonetically transcribe) the patients imitations.

1. _____
_____
2. _____
_____
3. _____
_____
4. _____
_____

V. CONNECTED SPEECH SAMPLE

Have the patient read "My Grandfather" or another standard reading passage and rate the following questions.

	Yes	No	Degree
1. Are vowels and consonants produced clearly?	☐	☐	_____
2. Is the patient's rate of speech too slow? Or is it too fast?	☐	☐	_____
3. Does the patient show inappropriate silent intervals between words?	☐	☐	_____
4. Does the patient show hypernasality?	☐	☐	_____
5. Is nasal emission present?	☐	☐	_____
6. Does the patient vary loudness normally?	☐	☐	_____
7. If not, is there evidence of monoloudness?	☐	☐	_____
8. Is there evidence of tremor in the patient's voice?	☐	☐	_____
9. Does the patient show abnormal pitch variations?	☐	☐	_____
10. Does the patient's voice have a harsh vocal quality?	☐	☐	_____
11. Does the patient's voice have a strained-strangled vocal quality?	☐	☐	_____
12. Does the patient's voice have a breathy vocal quality?	☐	☐	_____
13. Does the patient speak in abnormally short phrases?	☐	☐	_____

	Yes	No	Degree
14. Are there moments of involuntary inhalation or exhalation?	☐	☐	_____
15. Is inhalatory stridor present?	☐	☐	_____
16. Does the patient use normal stress on the appropriate syllables or words?	☐	☐	_____
17. If not, is there a reduction in normal stress?	☐	☐	_____
18. Or is there excess and equal stress?	☐	☐	_____

C H A P T E R

3

The Motor System

The parts of the nervous system that control voluntary movement are known collectively as the motor system. Understanding how this system works is an important part of being an effective diagnostician of motor speech disorders. Familiarity with the workings of upper and lower motor neurons, the basal ganglia and the cerebellum, and the pyramidal and the extrapyramidal systems is essential in making the correct diagnosis of a motor speech disorder and in designing appropriate treatment plans. This chapter provides an overview of the motor system to lay the foundation for the more specific investigations of the motor speech disorders presented in later chapters.

The motor system is what allows thought to be turned into movement, whether it is moving a hand, a leg, or the tongue. By any measure, the motor system is extremely complex. The nerve cells of the motor system are arranged into many different pathways, with each pathway performing different functions. Some parts of the motor system work at a conscious level, others at a subconscious level. The system's scope also is impressive. It ranges from very highest cognitive centers of the brain down to the body's simplest muscles. A properly functioning motor system allows movements of the fingers, vocal folds, feet, and eyebrows, all at the same time and in a coordinated manner. But, when a portion of it is damaged, the result can be a debilitating movement disorder. The type of disorder is dependent on the location and extent of the damage to the motor system. For example, lesions in a region of the brain called the basal ganglia can result in involuntary movements that seriously interfere with an individual's voluntary attempts to speak, walk, or do any number of other things. Because of this relationship between the type of disorder and the site of damage, it is important to understand the basics of the motor system.

COMPONENTS OF THE NERVOUS SYSTEM

The motor system is actually one of several subdivisions of the nervous system. Consequently, any discussion of the motor system would be difficult, if not impossible, without a basic understanding of the nervous system. Because of the link between the nervous and motor system, the first portion of this chapter reviews the fundamental structures of the nervous system.

The nervous system is organized into the central and peripheral nervous systems (Figure 3–1). The **central nervous system** (CNS) consists of the brain and the spinal cord. The **peripheral nervous system** (PNS) is composed of 12 pairs of cranial nerves and 31 pairs of spinal

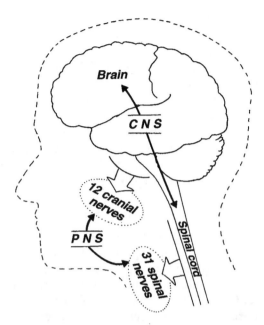

Figure 3–1. The central nervous system consists of the brain and spinal cord. The peripheral nervous system contains the 12 cranial nerves and the 31 spinal nerves. (From *The Speech Sciences* [p. 241], by R. Kent, 1997, San Diego: Singular Publishing Group, Inc. Copyright 1997 by Singular Publishing Group, Inc. Reprinted with permission.)

nerves. The cranial nerves are so named because they project from parts of the CNS that are within the cranium (i.e., inside the skull). They innervate many organs and muscles of the head, neck, thorax, and abdomen. In contrast, the spinal nerves branch from the spinal cord and innervate most of the other muscles of the body, including the chest, arms, and legs.

Brain

Of course, the brain is the key component of the nervous system. It is the most complex part of the nervous system. Almost all activity in the nervous system originates in or is ultimately processed by the brain. Voluntary motor commands to the muscles originate in the brain. The brain also receives sensory information from the body and controls the cognitive functions, including reasoning, memory, language, imagining, and so forth.

Compared to most other animals, humans have large brains relative to body size. The normal adult brain weighs about 2.5 to 3.5 lbs. It has an amazingly complex number of interconnections among its various parts, as well as with the other portions of the nervous system. The following paragraphs review the parts of the brain that are most relevant to understanding the motor system.

Cerebrum

The brain is divided into the **cerebrum, brainstem,** and **cerebellum** (Figure 3–2). The largest and most prominent of these is the cerebrum. It is split into two hemispheres by the longitudinal fissure, which runs front to back along the middle of the brain. The cerebrum is organized into four different areas called lobes. The **frontal lobe** is located on the anterior (front) portion of the cerebrum. The **temporal lobe** lies on the lower sides of the cerebrum. The **parietal lobe** is found on the upper sides of the cerebrum behind the frontal lobe. Lastly, the **occipital lobe** is on the rear-most portion of the cerebrum, behind the parietal and temporal lobes. The most obvious feature of the cerebrum is its deep convolutions. Each convolution is called a **gyrus** (plural = gyri), and the groove between the gyri is called a **sulcus** (plural = sulci).

The gyri and sulci of the cerebrum create several significant landmarks that will be referred to frequently in this textbook (Figure 3–3). The first of these is the **lateral sulcus,** certainly the most prominent sulcus on the cerebrum. It runs horizontally along the lateral sides of each hemisphere and separates the temporal lobe from the frontal lobe. Another landmark is the **central sulcus,** probably the second most prominent sulcus on the cerebrum. It is located near the center of the lateral sides of each hemisphere (hence its name) and extends vertically from the very top of the hemisphere down to the lateral sulcus.

The gyrus immediately in front of the central sulcus is known variously as the **precentral gyrus,** the **primary motor cortex,** or the **motor strip.** The nerve cells located in this gyrus play a very important role in controlling the voluntary movements of the body. The gyrus just behind the central sulcus is called either the postcentral gyrus, the primary sensory cortex, or the sensory strip. Here, the higher centers of the brain receive sensory information from the body via the PNS and other portions of the CNS.

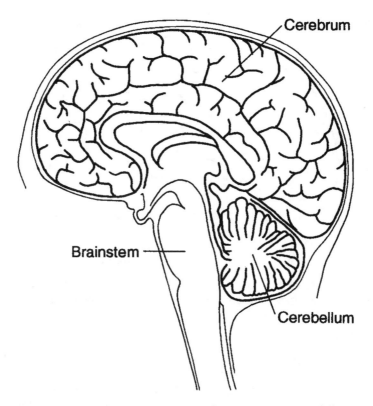

Figure 3–2. The brain consists of the cerebrum, brainstem, and cerebellum. (From *Anatomy and Physiology for Speech, Language, and Hearing* [p. 383], by J. Seikel, D. King, and D. Drumright, 1997, San Diego: Singular Publishing Group, Inc. Copyright 1997 by Singular Publishing Group, Inc. Reprinted with permission.)

The surface of the cerebrum is called the **cerebral cortex**. It varies between 2 mm and 5 mm in thickness and is composed of six different layers of nervous system cells. In its entirety, the cortex contains about 15 billion nerve cells (neurons). The cortex is gray in color and is often described as being the "gray matter" of the brain. Only about one third of the cortex is visible because of the cerebrum's many convolutions; the other two thirds are hidden between the many sulci. If laid flat, the total surface area of the cortex would be approximately 340 square inches. The cortex is one of the most important parts of the nervous system. In this cortical layer of nerve cells, the higher cognitive activi-

Precentral Gyrus

Postcentral Gyrus

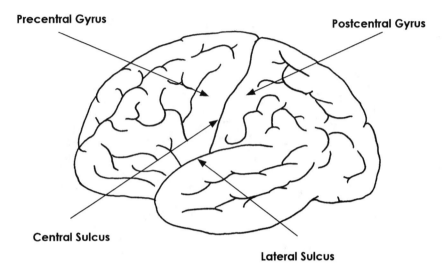

Central Sulcus

Lateral Sulcus

Figure 3–3. Four of the most prominent landmarks on the lateral surface of the brain are the lateral and central sulci and the precentral and postcentral gyri.

ties, such as language, motor planning, problem solving, and much sensory perception, are performed. Because it is so thin, the cortex makes up only a small percentage of the cerebrum's total size. Most of the cerebrum is actually composed of large groupings of white matter located below the cortex. This white matter consists of nerve cell axons that course to and from other parts of the CNS. The white color is from the fatty myelin that covers the axons. More information about axons and myelin is presented shortly.

Brainstem

The brainstem is divided (from top to bottom) into the **midbrain, pons, and medulla** (Figure 3–4). It sits between the cerebrum and the spinal cord. The brainstem's importance is threefold. First, it acts as a passageway for the descending and ascending neural tracts that travel between the cerebrum and spinal cord. Second, it controls certain integrative and reflexive actions, such as respiration, consciousness, and some parts of the cardiovascular system functions. Third, it contains the places where the cranial nerves project out from the CNS, which is probably the most important with regard to the motor speech system. It is the cranial nerves that convey motor impulses from the CNS to the muscles of the larynx,

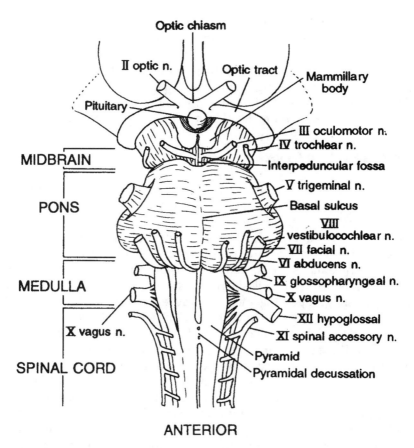

Figure 3–4. The brainstem is divided into the midbrain, pons, and medulla. This figure also illustrates the roots of the cranial nerves. (From *Anatomy and Physiology for Speech, Language, and Hearing* [p. 412], by J. Seikel, D. King, and D. Drumright, 1997, San Diego: Singular Publishing Group, Inc. Copyright 1997 by Singular Publishing Group, Inc. Reprinted with permission.)

face, tongue, pharynx, and velum. The cranial nerves are attached to the brainstem at points called the **cranial nerve nuclei**.

Cerebellum

The cerebellum is shaped somewhat like the cerebrum but is much smaller. It is attached to the back of the brainstem, where it makes neural connections with the cerebral cortex and numerous other parts of the

CNS. The most important function of the cerebellum is to coordinate voluntary movements, so muscles contract with the correct amount of force and at the appropriate times. Cerebellar damage can cause significant deficits in the performance of both gross and skilled motor actions. Movements such as walking, writing, and speech can become uncertain and awkward when the cerebellum is not functioning properly. The cerebellum is examined in more detail later in this chapter and in Chapter 7.

Nervous System Cells

The nervous system contains many different types of cells. The most important are the **neurons** (Figure 3–5). They are the cells that transmit the electrochemical signals that control nearly every function of the body. Estimates of the number of neurons in the human body range from 50 to 100 billion. Neurons have three primary components. The first is the **cell body**, which contains the nucleus responsible for the cell's vital metabolic functions. The cell bodies of neurons are gray in color. When many cell bodies are grouped together, they cause the distinctive grayish tint that is visible in many structures in the CNS, such as the cortex and the central portion of the spinal cord. **Dendrites** are the second component of neurons. These are the many short processes that extend from the cell body. Dendrites receive electrochemical impulses from other neurons or from sensory organs. The third component is the **axon**, the single long extension from the cell body. Axons conduct neural impulses away from the cell body and transfer the impulses to muscles, glands, or other neurons. The end of an axon may have many small branches called terminal ramifications, or terminal boutons, which allow one axon to communicate with many additional neurons. An axon also may have longer branches called collaterals, further extending the influence of a neuron to other parts of the nervous system.

Most axons are covered by **myelin,** a white, lipid-protein membrane that covers the length of the axon. Myelin insulates a neuron's electrochemical impulses from the surrounding tissues and fluids, which would otherwise degrade the strength of an impulse as it travels the length of the axon. Myelin acts very much like the insulation on household electrical wiring to prevent the leakage of electrical energy.

Types of Neurons

Neurons are categorized by their shape and size. Some neurons have their cell body in the middle of the axon; others have it to the side of the axon. Some have very large cell bodies; others do not. Some neurons have axons that are only a fraction of a millimeter long; others

Dendrites

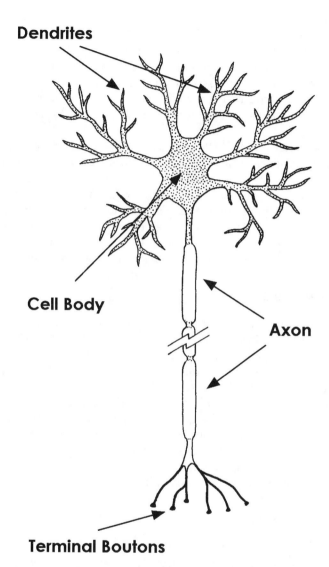

Cell Body

Axon

Terminal Boutons

Figure 3–5. A neuron contains many dendrites, a cell body, and a single axon. (From *Anatomy and Physiology for Speech, Language, and Hearing* [p. 389], by J. Seikel, D. King, and D. Drumright, 1997, San Diego: Singular Publishing Group, Inc. Copyright 1997 by Singular Publishing Group, Inc. Reprinted with permission.)

have axons up to a meter in length. In addition, neurons are classified by the types of information they carry. **Motor neurons** transmit neural impulses that cause contractions in muscles (and thereby cause movement). **Sensory neurons** carry information related to sensory stimuli. **Interneurons** link neurons with other neurons. Interneurons are the most common type of neuron. Because they form connections with many other neurons, interneurons play an important role in controlling movement.

Yet another distinction between neurons is the direction in which they convey neural impulses. Neurons that transmit their impulses away from the CNS are called **efferent neurons.** Those sending their impulses toward the CNS are called **afferent neurons.** In general, motor neurons are efferent, and sensory neurons are afferent. It is not unusual to use these terms to describe the flow of neural information from one area of the nervous system to another. For instance, the cortex may be said to receive afferent input from sensory neurons.

Other Nervous System Cells

Although neurons are the most important cells of the nervous system, they are certainly not the only ones, nor are they the most numerous. The other cells in the nervous system are called **glial cells** (or the neuroglia). They include **Schwann cells,** which provide the myelin sheath around axons in the PNS; **microglia,** which act as scavengers and remove dead cells and other waste; **oligodendroglia,** which form myelin around axons in the CNS; and **astrocytes,** which make up the connective tissue of the CNS. It is believed that there are 10 times as many glial cells as neurons and that they make up more than half the volume of the nervous system. Glial cells play a vital supporting role in the functioning of the nervous system.

Tracts and Nerves

Throughout the nervous system, axons are usually found coursing through the body in bundles. The axons in these bundles are often functionally related to each other. For example, there is a prominent bundle of motor neuron axons that travel together from the cortex to the spinal cord, all transmitting motor impulses. Another example is the bundle of sensory neuron axons extending from the retina of the eye to the visual centers of the brain. When bundles of axons such as these are found in the CNS, they are most often called **tracts.** When found in the PNS, they are called **nerves.** The bundles of axons in the prior two examples are properly called the corticospinal tract and the optic nerve. Note that the wording of the term *corticospinal* indicates the direction in which neural impulses travel within this tract. In this example, the flow is from the cortex (*cortico*) to the spinal cord (*spinal*).

Transmission of Neural Impulses

Stated simply, the function of a neuron is to transmit neural impulses from one part of the nervous system to another. A neuron accomplishes this by conducting a small electrochemical charge along the length of its axon. When this charge reaches the axon's terminal ramifications, small amounts of a substance called a **neurotransmitter** are released from these end points. The neurotransmitter crosses a microscopic gap (the **synaptic cleft**) between the active neuron and an adjoining neuron (Figure 3–6). Some neurotransmitters are excitatory in function, meaning they increase the probability of an electrochemical impulse being stimulated in the adjoining neuron. Other neurotransmitters are inhibitory and act to decrease the probability of an impulse occurring in the adjoining neuron. If enough of an excitatory neurotransmitter is received in specialized receptors in the adjoining neuron, an electrochemical impulse will be initiated in this neuron. In contrast, if too much an inhibitory neurotransmitter is present, the impulse will not be transmitted to the adjoining neuron. **Acetylcholine** and **dopamine** are two neurotransmitters that are important in the motor system.

It is misleading, however, to concentrate too narrowly on the functioning of just a few neurons when describing the transmission of neural impulses. The true picture is really much, much more complicated. There are two important points to remember when visualizing how neurons communicate. The first is that a single neuron may have synaptic connections with the terminal ramifications or collaterals of *many* different axons. In fact, a typical neuron has several thousand synaptic connections with other neurons. Consequently, a single neuron may synapse with some axons that are producing excitatory neurotransmitters and with others producing inhibitory neurotransmitters.

This leads to the second important point. A receiving neuron will fire its own electrochemical impulse only when a certain threshold of excitation is reached and then only if the amounts of excitatory neurotransmitters exceed the influence of inhibitory neurotransmitters. The nervous system depends on this complex interplay of excitatory and inhibitory neurotransmitters to effectively convey neural impulses. When this interplay is not kept in balance, the results can be serious. In the motor system an imbalance between excitatory and inhibitory neu-

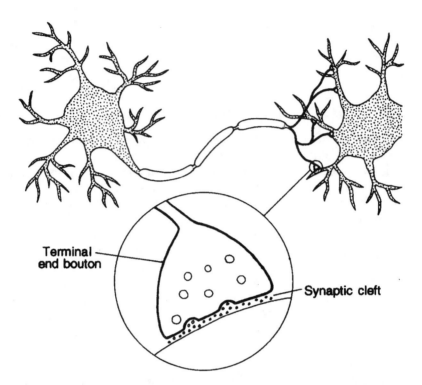

Figure 3–6. Neurons communicate with each other across microscopic gaps called synaptic clefts. (Adapted from *Anatomy and Physiology for Speech, Language, and Hearing* [p. 390], by J. Seikel, D. King, and D. Drumright, 1997, San Diego: Singular Publishing Group, Inc. Copyright 1997 by Singular Publishing Group, Inc. Reprinted with permission.)

rotransmitters may be a cause of spasticity. For example, if a stroke or physical trauma damages a tract of inhibitory motor neurons, its neurons will not be able to contribute their inhibitory neurotransmitters to their synaptic connections with other motor neurons. In this case, there will be a relatively disproportionate amount of excitatory neurotransmitters affecting those other neurons. The result will be excessive contractions of the muscles innervated by those highly excited neurons that did not receive the counterbalancing inhibitory neurotransmitters. The causes of spasticity are explored in more detail in later sections of this book.

Summary of Motor System Components

- The nervous system is divided into the CNS and the PNS. The CNS includes the brain and the spinal cord. The PNS includes the spinal and cranial nerves.
- The brain is organized into the cerebrum, brainstem, and cerebellum. The cerebrum is divided into four lobes: frontal, temporal, parietal, and occipital.
- The most important cells of the nervous system are neurons. They are means by which neural impulses are transmitted from one part of the nervous system to another.

STRUCTURE AND FUNCTION
OF THE MOTOR SYSTEM

The remainder of this chapter concentrates on the structure and function of the motor system. The following pages present a model of how the motor system is organized and how its components interact during movement. Admittedly, it is a simplified model. Some components of the motor system have been combined, others glossed over, and a few omitted. For example, the influence of sensory information on movement is not examined in detail, nor are the limbic system's contributions included. (The limbic system is a subcortical area of the brain influencing emotion, memory, learning, and related behaviors.) Refer to Figure 3–7 frequently while reading the following paragraphs because each box in the diagram is detailed individually. The boxes represent parts of the motor system, and the arrows indicate the flow of neural information from one part to another.

Desire to Move

The starting place for any voluntary movement is having the desire to move. It is the first step in picking up an object, walking, standing, phonating, or any of a hundred other actions that are performed everyday. Taking that desire and turning it into a movement is something most individuals can do quite easily. It seems like a simple task. In reality, however, it is exceedingly complex. In fact, *it is not understood how the brain transforms the desire to move into a sequence of motor neuron firing*. The nature of the neurological "spark" that begins the whole

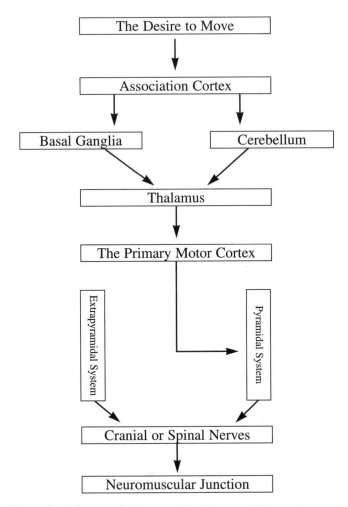

Figure 3–7. A simplified schematic diagram of the motor system.

process of planning a movement is unknown. One textbook jokingly described it as a small person inside the brain pulling the appropriate strings when an individual wants to move.

Currently, it can only be assumed that thought somehow triggers the firing of the correct neurons that lead to a desired movement. Although it is not known how the desire to move initiates movement, many of the subsequent steps in the motor system are better understood. It is known, for example, that there is a significant increase in metabolic activity over large bilateral areas of the cortex, called the association cortex, about 800 ms before a voluntary movement is actually performed.

Consequently, it is believed that the association cortex plays an especially important role in the initial planning of voluntary movements.

Primary and Association Cortex

A discussion of the association cortex needs to be preceded by an examination of the primary cortex. This is because the association cortex receives much of its sensory input from the primary cortex. The **primary cortex** comprises the parts of the cerebrum that are dedicated to the analysis of a single type of neural input. Individually, these areas are known as the primary auditory cortex, primary visual cortex, primary sensory cortex, and primary motor cortex (Figure 3–8). The first three are responsible for the initial cortical processing of auditory, visual, and somatosensory (i.e., bodily sensation) information, respectively. The processing performed in these areas is relatively basic compared to the more complex analysis performed in higher centers of the brain. For example, the **primary auditory cortex**, which is located on the uppermost portion of the temporal lobe, is thought to analyze tone patterns and sound properties. It also may help in the localization of sounds. The more sophisticated analyses of sound are completed in other areas of the cortex.

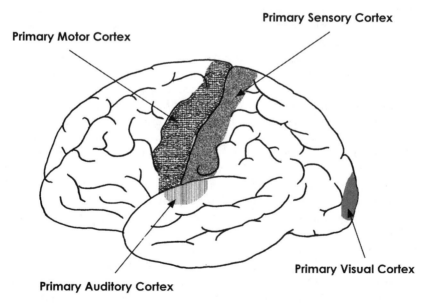

Figure 3–8. The four areas of the primary cortex.

The **primary visual cortex** is located at the most posterior end of the occipital lobe. It is thought to perform a preliminary analysis of depth and perhaps integration of visual information from both eyes. Damage to this area can result in the loss of conscious awareness of visual stimulation.

The **primary sensory cortex** is located on the postcentral gyrus. This is where the cortex receives the first neural input about bodily sensation. The analysis includes sensations of pressure, temperature, touch, and pain.

These three primary cortex areas are similar in that they are the first cortical areas to analyze sensory information. The primary motor cortex, which is located on the precentral gyrus, works in a comparable but reversed manner. It receives planned motor impulses from cortical and subcortical areas of the brain (to be discussed shortly) and sends those impulses down through the brainstem and spinal cord, where they are eventually sent to the muscles. An important point to remember is that most planning for movement does *not* originate in the primary motor cortex. It is thought that the initial planning of a movement is formulated elsewhere in the brain, primarily in the association cortex.

The **association cortex** is the area of the cortex that, in conjunction with other parts of the brain, "makes sense" of the sensory impulses that have been initially analyzed by the primary cortex. The association cortex, however, is not a single region of the brain. It is actually distributed over four areas of the cortex. These four areas are known as the temporal association area, parietal association area, frontal association area, and occipital association area (Figure 3–9). Although each area is covered individually in the following paragraphs, it would be a mistake to think of them as independent centers for specific types of processing. The association areas of the cortex are heavily interconnected with many other parts of the brain, and they function together in various combinations during mental tasks. The parietal association area, for example, has neural connections with at least eight other cortical areas, including the primary sensory cortex, the temporal association area, and the frontal association area. Given these many cortical connections (and their numerous connections with subcortical structures), it is not surprising to find that the association cortex operates in a highly integrated fashion.

The **temporal association area** covers much of the upper and central parts of the temporal lobe. It has neural connections with the frontal association area, the primary auditory cortex, certain visual processing regions along the bottom rear edge of the temporal lobe, and subcortical areas involved with memory. The workings of the temporal association area are diverse. It is involved with the recognition of complex visual stimuli, integrating auditory stimuli with other centers of

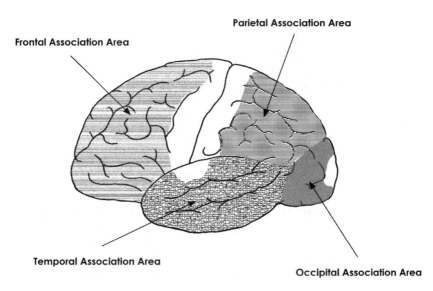

Figure 3–9. The four areas of the association cortex.

the brain, and the formation of memories. Damage to this area can result in visual agnosia, amnesia, and high levels of distractibility.

The **frontal association area** is found on the forward-most half of the frontal lobe. This area of the brain is sometimes called the prefrontal cortex to differentiate it from the cortical motor areas that are located on the frontal lobes (see Figure 3–9). The frontal association area has many neural connections with all the lobes of the cerebrum. Because of these numerous pathways, this area has access to all the sensory centers of the brain. The frontal association area also receives information on emotion and motivation from subcortical structures. Through the integration of this information, *the frontal association area undoubtedly plays an important role in initiating and planning of volitional movements*. Bilateral damage to this area can result in decreased spontaneity and initiative, shortened attention span, and difficulties with abstract problem solving.

The **parietal association area** is located between the primary sensory cortex and the occipital lobe. This area is responsible for integrating bodily sensations with visual information. In addition, it has many neural connections with the prefrontal and motor areas of the frontal lobe. As part of the motor system, *the parietal association area plays an important role in the control of visually guided movements (e.g., hand-eye coordination)*. Damage here can cause impairments in manipulating objects, sensory neglect of half the body, and certain reading and writing deficits.

The **visual association area** is a band of the cortex that runs between the primary visual cortex and the parietal and temporal lobes. It has many connections with the primary visual cortex, through which it receives visual sensory impulses. Its main function is to perform very complex analyses of visual impulses from the primary visual cortex. *The contributions of the visual association cortex to the motor system include its input to the parietal association area regarding visually guided movements.* Although selective damage to the visual association area is rare, it can result in several unusual disorders. One is motion blindness. In this condition, affected individuals have difficulty perceiving the movement of objects. For instance, running water will appear to be frozen in a fixed position; people walking in a room will seem to suddenly appear and disappear; an oncoming train will first seem to be far away and then suddenly it will be very close. Other disorders associated with visual association area damage are color blindness and prosopagnosia (the inability to recognize familiar faces).

In a process that is not well understood, these four cortical association areas, along with other parts of the brain, are able to take that nebulous "desire to move" and turn it into a planned pattern of muscular contractions. At this early stage of creating a movement, however, the planned contractions are believed to be rough and exaggerated approximations of what is really needed to successfully accomplish the desired movement. Further processing of the planned movement is required. That is where the basal ganglia, cerebellum, and thalamus enter the picture. The association cortex sends this rough sequence of motor impulses down to these subcortical structures for further processing.

Basal Ganglia and Cerebellum

The association cortex sends its neural signals of an intended motor movement to both the basal ganglia and the cerebellum. These two structures seem to have equally important, yet different effects on planned movements. Each has its own separate looping neural circuit, often called control circuits. Through these circuits, the basal ganglia and cerebellum link the association cortex with the primary motor cortex. That is, they take the rough motor impulses from the association cortex, smooth them out, coordinate them, and then send them (via the thalamus) up to the primary motor cortex.

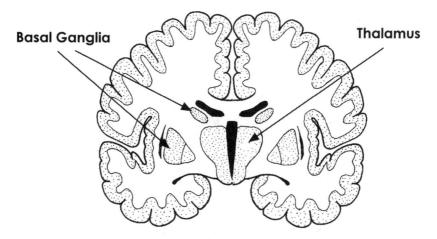

Basal Ganglia   **Thalamus**

Figure 3–10. A coronal section of the brain showing the positions of the basal ganglia and the thalamus. (Adapted from *Neuroscience of Communication* [p. 176], by D. Webster, 1999, San Diego: Singular Publishing Group, Inc. Copyright 1999 by Singular Publishing Group, Inc. Reprinted with permission.)

Basal Ganglia

The term basal ganglia is a collective name for three large subcortical structures located near the lateral ventricles (Figure 3–10). Individually, they are called the **caudate nucleus**, the **putamen**, and the **globus pallidus**. All three are interconnected with assorted neural fibers. The caudate nucleus and putamen are known together as the **striatum**. Because they are dense with gray matter (i.e., the cell bodies of neurons), they are quite distinct visually from the surrounding white matter. The basal ganglia contain an extremely complex network of neural pathways and have connections with many cortical and subcortical areas. They receive neural information from almost all areas of the cortex. Much of the neural output from the basal ganglia is sent to the thalamus (another subcortical gray matter structure that is discussed shortly).

The workings of the basal ganglia are very intricate and are not completely understood. However, their influence on movement is clear. *The basal ganglia are believed to be especially important in the planning of slow, continuous movements.* They are quite active during those types of movements and, in turn, are mostly inactive during rapid back and forth movements.

Several other subcortical gray matter structures influence the basal ganglia. One of them is the **substantia nigra** (Figure 3–11). It is connect-

Basal Ganglia

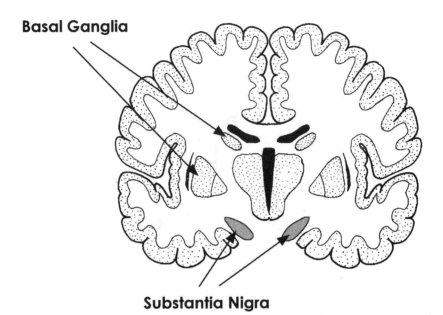

Substantia Nigra

Figure 3–11. A coronal section of the brain showing the position of the substantia nigra in relation to the basal ganglia. (Adapted from *Neuroscience of Communication* [p. 176], by D. Webster, 1999, San Diego: Singular Publishing Group, Inc. Copyright 1999 by Singular Publishing Group, Inc. Adapted with permission.)

ed to the striatum via its own neural circuit. The neural tract from the substantia nigra to the striatum contains a large number of neurons that produce the neurotransmitter dopamine. Many neurons of the striatum are dependent on dopamine for proper functioning. If the levels of dopamine from the substantia nigra are lowered in the striatum, the results may include muscular rigidity, tremor, gait disturbances, and difficulty initiating movement. This decrease in dopamine in the striatum can occur either as part of a disease process (e.g., Parkinson's disease) or can be acquired through other means, such an adverse effect of antipsychotic drugs that block the production of dopamine. The motor speech disorder associated with parkinsonism is called **hypokinetic dysarthria**. This type of dysarthria is discussed in Chapter 8.

Another class of movement disorders, known as **hyperkinetic disorders,** also is identified with damage to the basal ganglia. The symptoms of these disorders can be dramatically different from the tight, restricted movements seen in parkinsonian-type disorders. Huntington disease (also known as Huntington chorea) is a good example of a hyperkinetic movement disorder. It is a fatal, inherited disease that results in the progressive loss of neurons in the striatum and other areas of the brain. The symptoms of the disorder include rapid, involuntary movements of the extremities, face, and tongue. As the disease progresses, the movements increase in intensity and may begin to affect the muscles of the torso. Dementia and behavioral problems eventually become evident as well. The movements of the hands, arms, and legs in an individual with Huntington disease have sometimes been described as "dancelike" and "graceful." Although accurate to some extent, such descriptions minimize the debilitating effects these involuntary movements have on an individual's voluntary movements. The motor speech disorder found in Huntingtons disease and similar disorders is called **hyperkinetic dysarthria**, which is examined in Chapter 9.

Cerebellum

The cerebellum helps to regulate muscle tone, maintain balance, and coordinate skilled motor movements. It is attached to the back of the brainstem and lies just below the occipital lobe of the cerebrum (Figure 3–12). Its name, which literally means "little cerebrum," comes from early anatomists, who thought it was an additional, smaller brain. This erroneous conclusion is understandable as the cerebrum and cerebellum have a similar outward appearance. Like the cerebrum, the cerebellum has two hemispheres that are divided by a (small) fissure. Its surface also contains many convolutions and grooves—more, in fact, than are found on the cerebrum. Because of these numerous convolutions, the cerebellum has a surface area that is nearly 75% of that in the cerebral cortex.

   Like the basal ganglia, the cerebellum also receives neural impulses of intended motor movements from the association cortex. In addition, it receives sensory input from the vestibular labyrinth of the inner ear and from visual, tactile, auditory, and proprioceptive sensory receptors located throughout the body, all of which give the cerebellum access to information about the body's balance, position, and posture. It is thought that the cerebellum takes the preliminary motor impulses from the association cortex and integrates them with the sensory information available to it. *The cerebellum adjusts and refines the motor impulses according to the body's immediate circumstances* and sends these processed motor signals to the primary motor cortex via the thalamus. However, not all of the motor output from the cerebellum goes to the thalamus. It also has efferent neural tracts that indirectly synapse with

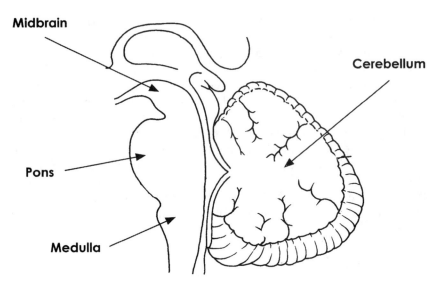

Midbrain

Cerebellum

Pons

Medulla

Figure 3–12. The cerebellum is attached to the posterior of the brainstem, which consists of the midbrain, pons, and medulla. (Adapted from *Anatomy and Physiology for Speech, Language, and Hearing* [p. 473], by J. Seikel, D. King, and D. Drumright, 1997, San Diego: Singular Publishing Group, Inc. Copyright 1997 by Singular Publishing Group, Inc. Adapted with permission.)

descending extrapyramidal tracts (to be discussed shortly). Through these connections with the extrapyramidal motor neurons, the cerebellum has relatively direct influence on such motor activities as walking and maintaining posture.

Because of its many afferent and efferent connections with diverse parts of the nervous system, damage to the cerebellum can result in a variety of disorders. One of these is **ataxia,** which is a disturbance in the speed, range, and direction of movements. The muscle groups near the shoulders and pelvis in particular may be affected. The gait of an individual with ataxia is wide-based, lurching, and stumbling. It is often described as having a "drunken" character. **Intention tremor** also is found in lesions of the cerebellar hemispheres. This type of tremor is observed only during the performance of voluntary movements, such as reaching for a glass of water. It is not present while an individual is at rest. Other disorders include involuntary oscillatory movements of the eyes (nystagmus), increased or decreased muscle tone, and disturbances of equilibrium. The motor speech disorder usually associated with cerebellar lesions is **ataxic dysarthria**, which is discussed in Chapter 7.

Thalamus

The thalamus is yet another important subcortical gray matter structure. It is located behind the basal ganglia and to the lateral sides of the third ventricle (Figure 3–13). The thalamus has been described as the doorway through which subcortical systems of the nervous system communicate with the cerebral cortex. It receives neural inputs of planned motor movements from both the basal ganglia and the cerebellum. Exactly what it does with these signals is not precisely understood. It is known, however, that the thalamus has a vast amount of somatosensory information available to it. Practically every sensory

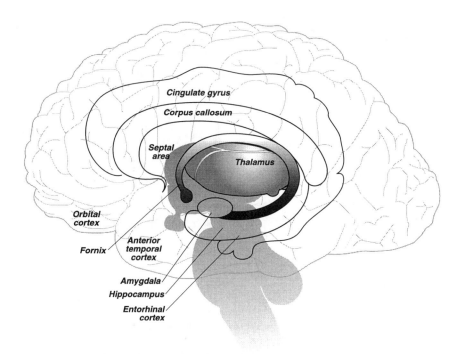

Figure 3–13. A lateral view of the thalamus in relation to the cerebrum. (Adapted from *The Speech Sciences* [p. 255], by R. Kent, 1997, San Diego: Singular Publishing Group, Inc. Copyright 1997 by Singular Publishing Group, Inc. Adapted with permission.)

impulse from the body passes through the thalamus on its way to the cortex. *It is believed that the thalamus uses this sensory information to further refine the motor impulses from the basal ganglia and cerebellum.*

Primary Motor Cortex

The primary motor cortex receives the neural motor impulses that have been processed, smoothed, and coordinated by the basal ganglia, the cerebellum, and thalamus. The neurons in the primary motor cortex have axons that are among the longest in the body. Many extend all the way from the cortex to the lower portions of the spinal cord. These axons make up much of the descending motor tract called the pyramidal system. Direct electrical stimulation of the primary motor cortex has shown that its neurons are arranged in an inverted body scheme (Figure 3–14). When

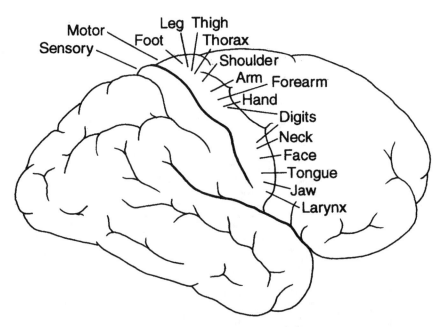

Figure 3–14. The neurons in the primary motor cortex are arranged in a inverted body scheme, with the neurons at the bottom of the gyrus being responsible for transmitting motor impulses to the neck and face muscles and the neurons at the top transmitting the impulses for the leg and foot muscles. (From *Anatomy and Physiology for Speech, Language, and Hearing* [p. 456], by J. Seikel, D. King, and D. Drumright, 1997, San Diego: Singular Publishing Group, Inc. Copyright 1997 by Singular Publishing Group, Inc. Reprinted with permission.)

neurons near the bottom of the precentral gyrus are stimulated with an electrical probe, contractions occur in the muscles of the head and neck muscles. In contrast, muscle contractions are observed in the leg and foot when neurons near the top of the gyrus are stimulated.

Direct electrical stimulation of the primary motor cortex also has revealed another important finding: stimulation never elicits a complex, coordinated motor movement. Only simple muscle contractions are observed. This implies that the primary motor cortex is not the designer of purposeful, sequenced movements. If it were, electrical stimulation of its neurons would result in some type of complex movement pattern. *The principal role of the primary motor cortex is thought to be: (a) to take voluntary movement patterns that are formulated elsewhere and (b) to transmit them to the cranial or spinal nerves via a tract of motor neurons called the pyramidal system.*

However, it is too simplistic to think of the primary motor cortex as just a relay station for incoming movement patterns. It also has the ability to integrate information from other cortical areas into a planned movement. The **premotor area** and **supplementary motor area** both provide additional input to the primary motor cortex just before a movement is initiated (Figure 3–15). These two cortical areas are located immediately anterior to the primary motor cortex, with the supplementary motor area extending over the top of the cerebral hemisphere and down into the longitudinal fissure. The neural signals contributed by these two areas are believed to exert further control over the final motor signals sent out by the primary motor cortex. The impulses from the premotor area seem to be especially important in visually guided movements, such as inserting a key in a lock. When this area is damaged, hand movements are notably clumsy. The influence of the supplementary motor area is a bit less definite. Neural signals from this area appear to facilitate the simultaneous use of both hands during complex sequences of movements.

Descending Motor Tracts

The descending motor tracts are the neural pathways carrying motor impulses that travel from the cortex to the brainstem and spinal cord. They are divided into two categories: the pyramidal system and extrapyramidal system. The functions of these two systems can be generalized by saying that *the **pyramidal system** is responsible for carrying the impulses that control voluntary, fine motor movements*, and *the **extrapyramidal system** transmits impulses that control the postural support needed by those fine motor movements.* For example, when someone

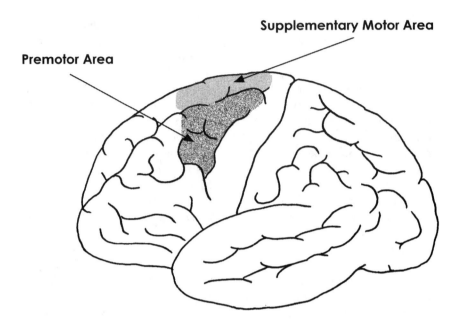

Premotor Area

Supplementary Motor Area

Figure 3–15. The premotor and supplementary motor areas play important roles in controlling and refining movements. The premotor area contributes to visually guided movements, and the supplementary motor area helps coordinate complex movements that involve the use of both hands.

is typing on a keyboard, it is the pyramidal system that carries the motor impulses that enable the person to make coordinated, independent finger movements on the keys. The extrapyramidal system, in turn, carries the impulses that keep the arms, shoulders, and back in a position that permit the fingers to move over the keyboard. Another generalization about these two systems is that the pyramidal system works at a conscious level, with the extrapyramidal system being more unconscious and automatic in its functions. As with any generalization, these are not absolutely true in every respect, but they do provide a good starting point for understanding the complex motor pathways that connect the higher centers of the brain to the muscles.

Pyramidal System

In the pyramidal system, most of the nerve fibers take a more or less direct path from the primary motor cortex to the brainstem or spinal cord, where they eventually synapse with cranial or spinal nerves. In fact, the pyramidal tract is sometimes called the direct activation system because of its relatively straight pathway from the cortex to the cranial and spinal nerves. Incidentally, the name pyramidal system comes from a point in the medulla (called the pyramids) where these descending fibers are compressed tightly together. By whatever name, this motor pathway is a key component of the motor system. Its fibers are divided into the corticospinal and corticobulbar tracts. The **corticospinal tract** is made up of axons that descend down from the cortex, through the internal capsule, the brainstem, and into the spinal cord (Figure 3–16). The axons terminate in the spinal cord, where many of them synapse with spinal nerves. The **corticobulbar tract** also is composed of axons descending from the cortex, but its axons terminate in the brainstem, where they synapse eventually with the cranial nerves. The term *bulbar* is a reference to an old name for the medulla, which once was known as *the bulb*. In sum, the pyramidal system consists of motor neurons that make a mostly direct course from the cortex to the spinal cord (corticospinal tract) or to the brainstem (corticobulbar tract).

Most axons of the pyramidal system have cell bodies that are located in the primary motor cortex. Some fibers of this system, however, also originate from the premotor cortex, the supplementary motor cortex, and the primary sensory cortex. Both corticospinal and corticobulbar fibers descend close to each other through the cerebrum. In the medulla, most corticospinal fibers cross the midline at a point called the pyramidal decussation and continue down on the opposite side into the spinal cord. Beginning in the midbrain and continuing through the rest of the brainstem, the corticobulbar fibers gradually separate from the corticospinal fibers.

Unlike the corticospinal fibers, the corticobulbar fibers do not all cross the midline. They are distributed in a complex bilateral pattern before they synapse with the cranial nerves (Figure 3–17), which results in bilateral cortical innervation for most cranial nerves. This means, for example, that a stroke affecting the corticobulbar fibers in the left hemisphere will not paralyze *most* muscles served by the cranial nerves. This is because both the right and left cranial nerves will still receive motor innervation from the undamaged right hemisphere. The cranial nerves serving the muscles of the larynx, pharynx, palate, upper face, and jaw all receive this bilateral innervation. Keep in mind, however, that the muscles of the lower face and tongue have primarily unilateral innervation. These two muscle groups could be notably affected by unilateral cortical damage. Cranial nerve innervation of the head and neck muscles is discussed in greater detail in the next chapter.

The pyramidal system is rudimental in such lower animals as mice and rats. In successively higher animals (dogs, monkeys, humans), it

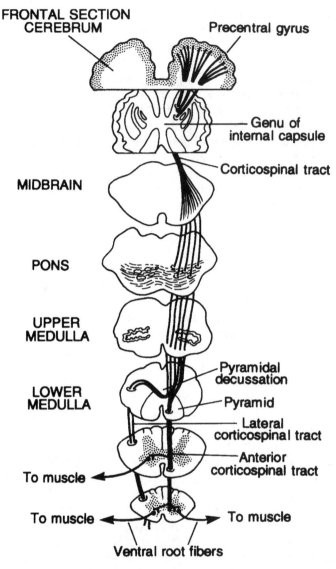

FRONTAL SECTION
CEREBRUM
Precentral gyrus

Genu of
internal capsule

Corticospinal tract

MIDBRAIN

PONS

UPPER
MEDULLA

LOWER
MEDULLA

Pyramidal
decussation

Pyramid

Lateral
corticospinal tract

Anterior
corticospinal tract

To muscle

To muscle

To muscle

Ventral root fibers

Figure 3–16. The corticospinal tract of the pyramidal system
provides a more or less direct connection between the primary motor cortex (precentral gyrus) and the spinal nerves. (From
Anatomy and Physiology for Speech, Language, and Hearing
[p. 407], by J. Seikel, D. King, and D. Drumright, 1997, San
Diego: Singular Publishing Group, Inc. Copyright 1997 by
Singular Publishing Group, Inc. Reprinted with permission.)

PRECENTRAL GYRUS
OF CEREBRAL CORTEX

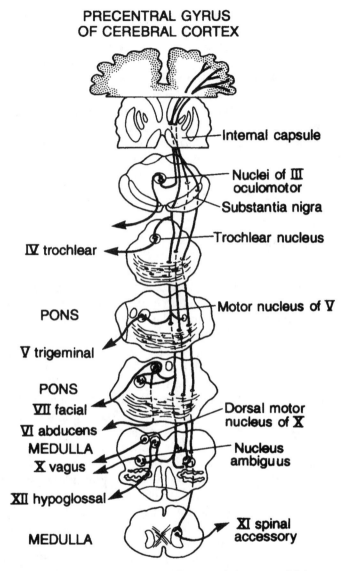

Figure 3–17. The corticobulbar tract of the pyramidal system connects the primary motor cortex (precentral gyrus) with most of the cranial nerves. (From *Anatomy and Physiology for Speech, Language, and Hearing* [p. 410], by J. Seikel, D. King, and D. Drumright, 1997, San Diego: Singular Publishing Group, Inc. Copyright 1997 by Singular Publishing Group, Inc. Reprinted with permission.)

becomes increasingly larger and sophisticated. Damage to these fibers usually results in muscle weakness and rapid fatigue. Patients with injuries to the pyramidal system also report that increased mental concentration is needed to perform motor tasks that were previously accomplished with ease. In the motor speech mechanism, unilateral damage to the pyramidal system results in a loss of fine motor movement in the articulators, a condition known as **unilateral upper motor neuron dysarthria** (see Chapter 6). However, the symptoms of pyramidal tract damage must be interpreted cautiously, because other neural tracts are located close to the pyramidal fibers as they course through the cerebrum and brainstem. Damage that affects the pyramidal tract will almost always affect these other tracts as well, with results that complicate the clinical picture.

Extrapyramidal System

The extrapyramidal system is composed of a number of different, interconnected descending motor pathways. The term *extrapyramidal* simply refers to the motor tracts that are not part of the pyramidal system ("extra" to the pyramidal system). Many neurophysiologists do not use the term extrapyramidal when referring to these additional motor tracts because they think it inadequately depicts their varied functions. Some prefer to call it the *indirect activation system*, thinking that this phrase better describes the system's complex, multiple interconnections. Others simply omit any single collective name and describe each descending motor pathway separately. While recognizing these objections, this textbook continues to use the term *extrapyramidal* for this system, because it is still used widely in clinical settings, and it does provide a broad, shorthand way to describe these motor tracts.

Four descending pathways of the extrapyramidal system will be discussed here: the rubrospinal tract, reticulospinal tract, vestibulospinal tract, and tectospinal tract. Remember that each of these is similar to the pyramidal system in that they are neural motor pathways between the higher levels of the nervous system and the cranial or spinal nerves. They are different in that they originate in the brainstem, not in the cortex. They also are different in that they have many connections with other regions of the brain as they proceed to the peripheral nerves. For example, the cerebral cortex, the basal ganglia, and the cerebellum all have neural connections to the extrapyramidal system, through which these higher levels of the brain are able to directly influence the actions of the muscles innervated by the extrapyramidal tracts.

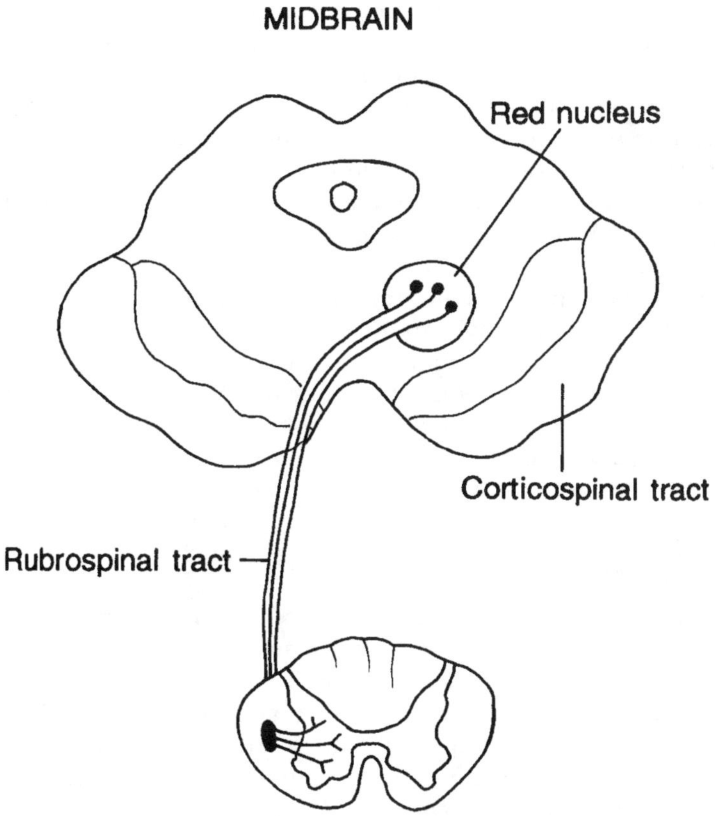

MIDBRAIN

Figure 3–18. The rubrospinal tract, which is one of tracts of the extrapyramidal system. (From *Anatomy and Physiology for Speech, Language, and Hearing* [p. 411], by J. Seikel, D. King, and D. Drumright, 1997, San Diego: Singular Publishing Group, Inc. Copyright 1997 by Singular Publishing Group, Inc. Reprinted with permission.)

The **rubrospinal tract** originates in a group of neurons in the brainstem called the red nucleus (Figure 3–18). Its nerve fibers cross the midline shortly after leaving the red nucleus and continue down to the spinal cord. Because many rubrospinal tract fibers are mixed with pyramidal fibers and have synaptic connections in many of the same areas, it is thought that this tract may assist the pyramidal system in controlling voluntary movements.

The **reticulospinal tract** originates in the reticular formation, which is a group of cells coursing through the midbrain, pons, and medulla. The reticular formation has several important functions. In addition to being part of the extrapyramidal motor system, it has controlling effects on an individual's level of consciousness, blood pressure, respiration, and attention. The fibers of the reticulospinal tract receive afferent input from many sources, including the motor and sensory cortex, the basal ganglia, the substantia nigra, and the red nucleus. Because of these varied inputs, the reticulospinal tract has an important influence on the spinal nerves. This tract is believed to be especially important in maintaining upright posture and the body's ability to turn toward external stimuli. It also may allow for some voluntary, gross motor movements, such as raising an arm or leg. Furthermore, the reticular formation and the reticulospinal tract contain "built in" reflexive motor patterns that can operate without higher nervous system input. For example, this tract enables some infants born without a cerebrum to perform certain basic movements such as sucking, stretching, and yawning.

The final two extrapyramidal tracts have little to do with motor speech production, so they are only mentioned briefly. The **vestibulospinal tract** originates in the vestibular apparatus of the inner ear, courses through the pons and medulla, and terminates in the spinal cord. It helps the body maintain posture and balance. The last tract is the **tectospinal tract**. Its fibers originate in the midbrain and end in the cervical portion of the spinal cord. This tract receives many afferent inputs from the eyes and the visual cortex and, consequently, plays an important role in keeping the eyes and the head oriented to external stimuli.

It is useful to think of the extrapyramidal system as operating in parallel with the pyramidal system. This means that while the pyramidal system is transmitting fine motor neural impulses to the cranial and spinal nerves, the extrapyramidal system is simultaneously controlling the muscles that provide the postural support needed to accomplish those fine motor movements. Taken as a whole, the postural muscles controlled by the extrapyramidal system include those of the torso and the larger muscle groups of the arms and legs. The extrapyramidal system's influence on the cranial nerves and muscles of the speech mechanism is not completely understood. It is known that neurons in the reticular formation (the origin of the reticulospinal tract) have many synaptic connections with the cranial nerves. Through those connections, *the extrapyramidal system influ-*

ences the reflexes, muscle tone, and probably some voluntary movements of the speech mechanism.

Cranial and Spinal Nerves

Before discussing cranial and spinal nerves, the difference between upper and lower motor neurons needs to be discussed. Various authors have used different criteria for defining upper motor neurons. For example, some say upper motor neurons are only those in the pyramidal system. Others state that the definition should include all the motor neurons in the CNS. This textbook will use this second definition. *Upper motor neurons are all the descending motor fibers coursing through the CNS, that eventually make a synaptic connection to the motor neurons in the PNS.* This includes the two pathways of the pyramidal system (the corticospinal and corticobulbar tracts) and the pathways of the extrapyramidal system (the rubrospinal, reticulospinal, vestibulospinal, and tectospinal tracts). To put it briefly, upper motor neurons are the motor fibers within the CNS. *Lower motor neurons, in contrast, are the motor neurons in the cranial and spinal nerves.* From a clinical standpoint, the distinction between these is important because damage to upper motor neurons results in symptoms that are usually quite different from those after damage to lower motor neurons. In general, upper motor neuron damage results in spasticity. The motor speech disorder associated with bilateral upper motor neuron damage is called **spastic dysarthria** (Chapter 5). Lower motor neuron damage results in muscle paralysis or paresis (weakness). **Flaccid dysarthria** (Chapter 4) is the result of damage to the lower motor neurons in those cranial nerves than innervate the muscles of speech production.

Cranial Nerve Nuclei

As stated previously, the cranial nerves are attached to the brainstem at points called the **cranial nerve nuclei**. As can be seen in Figure 3–19, a cranial nerve's sensory and motor fibers separately branch out from the brainstem. The cell bodies of the sensory neurons are gathered together outside of the brainstem in a bundle called a cranial ganglion. The cell bodies of the lower motor neurons are grouped inside the brainstem. It is in that area within the brainstem that the lower motor neurons in the cranial nerves synapse with upper motor neurons from the pyramidal and extrapyramidal systems. If the complex interaction of neurotransmitters from upper motor neurons reach a certain excitatory threshold, they will transmit their motor impulses to the cranial

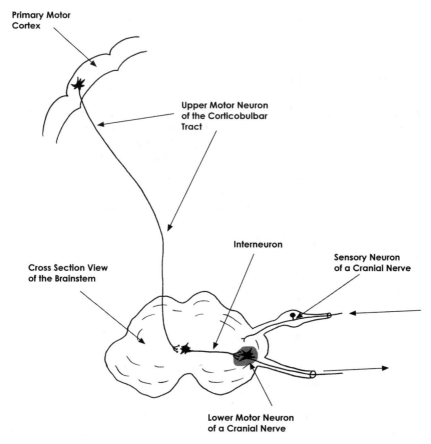

Figure 3–19. A typical neural pathway between the primary motor cortex and the lower motor neuron of a cranial nerve. The cell bodies of motor neurons in the cranial nerves are located within the brainstem at sites known as cranial nerve nuclei (shaded area).

nerve motor neuron, which then will transmit its own neural impulse directly to the muscle tissue it innervates.

Spinal Nerve Nuclei

The spinal nerves are attached to the spinal cord in a manner that is roughly similar to the cranial nerves and brainstem (Figure 3–20). The sensory and motor fibers branch from the spinal cord separately. As with the sensory fibers of the cranial nerves, there is a spinal ganglion

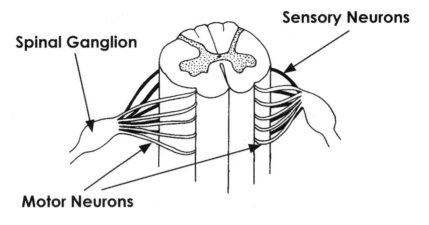

Figure 3–20. Motor neurons in spinal nerves branch off from the anterior portion of the spinal cord. (Adapted from *Anatomy and Physiology for Speech, Language, and Hearing* [p. 398], by J. Seikel, D. King, and D. Drumright, 1997, San Diego: Singular Publishing Group, Inc. Copyright 1997 by Singular Publishing Group, Inc. Adapted with permission.)

containing the cell bodies of the sensory neurons. Spinal sensory fibers attach to the spinal cord on its dorsal (back) surface. A cross-sectional view of the spinal cord (Figures 3–20 and 3–21) shows that the center of the spinal cord contains an H-shaped region of gray matter. This spinal gray matter is composed of neuron cell bodies that send their axons to other parts of the spinal cord or to the brain. The cell bodies of the lower motor neurons in the spinal nerves are located in the ventral (front) horn of the spinal gray matter. This is where the spinal lower motor neurons synapse with the pyramidal system, extrapyramidal system, and sensory neurons. From the ventral horn, the motor axons of the spinal nerves project out to the muscles they innervate. Again, the interplay of neurotransmitters from the upper motor and sensory neurons at their synaptic connections with the spinal lower motor neurons determines if a neural impulse will be transmitted to a muscle.

Neuromuscular Junction

Finally, the neural impulse arrives at the place where a muscle actually contracts to cause a movement. The **neuromuscular junction** is the

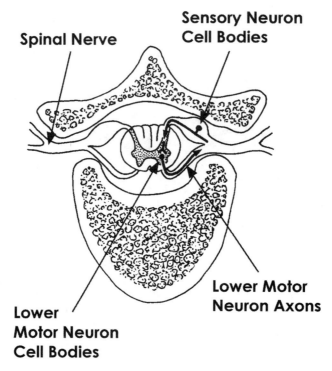

Spinal Nerve

Sensory Neuron Cell Bodies

Lower Motor Neuron Cell Bodies

Lower Motor Neuron Axons

Figure 3–21. The cell bodies of motor neurons in the spinal nerves are located in the ventral horns of the spinal cord gray matter. The cell bodies of sensory neurons in the spinal nerves are located just outside of the spinal cord. (Adapted from *Anatomy and Physiology for Speech, Language, and Hearing* [p. 399], by J. Seikel, D. King, and D. Drumright, 1997, San Diego: Singular Publishing Group, Inc. Copyright 1997 by Singular Publishing Group, Inc. Adapted with permission.)

point where the axons of lower motor neurons make synaptic connections with muscle cells (Figure 3–22). At the end of a motor neuron axon, there are many small terminal branches that synapse with the membrane of a muscle cell. Each one of these small branches makes a synaptic connection with only one muscle cell. When the neural impulse traveling down the axon reaches the terminal branch, the neurotransmitter acetylcholine is released by the axon into the microscopic gap between the axon and the muscle cell. This neurotransmitter binds to special receptors in the membrane of the muscle cell. When

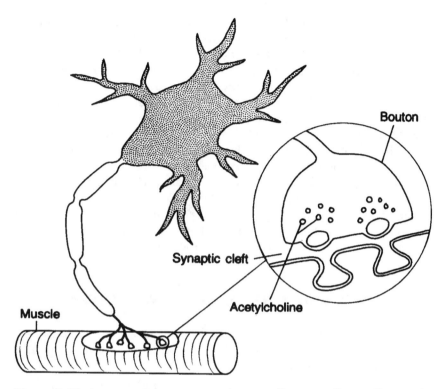

Figure 3–22. Lower motor neurons make synaptic connections with muscle tissue at the neuromuscular junction. (From *Anatomy and Physiology for Speech, Language, and Hearing* [p. 502], by J. Seikel, D. King, and D. Drumright, 1997, San Diego: Singular Publishing Group, Inc. Copyright 1997 by Singular Publishing Group, Inc. Reprinted with permission.)

enough acetylcholine is present in the muscle cell receptors, an electro-chemical impulse occurs throughout the cell. It is this final impulse in the muscle cell that causes the contraction of the muscle fiber.

With its numerous terminal branches, a single axon is able to cause contractions in many individual muscle cells. The actual number of muscle cells innervated by an axon varies according to the amount of fine motor control needed by a body part. A single axon may innervate many hundreds of individual muscle cells in large muscle groups or just a few cells in the muscles that perform intricate movements: it depends on how much control of the movement is necessary. In the thigh, for example, a neural impulse from one axon will cause the simultaneous contraction of many muscle cells, which is appropriate as the thigh is seldom called upon to make small, discrete movements. However, in the face or fingers, one axon will control only a handful of muscle fibers, resulting in greater cortical control over the contractions of those muscles. This difference in the number of muscle fibers innervated by a single axon is called the **innervation ratio**.

As stated at the beginning of this chapter, understanding the motor system is an important part of making the correct diagnosis of a motor speech disorder, as well as developing an appropriate treatment plan. If damage in any part of the motor system affects the muscles of speech production, the result can be a motor speech disorder. The particular motor speech disorder that occurs depends on which part of the motor system is damaged. Each of the upcoming chapters of this textbook examines one of the dysarthrias and apraxia of speech. Significant parts of the chapters are devoted to explaining how these disorders are linked to damage to specific parts of the motor system.

SUMMARY OF THE MOTOR SYSTEM

- The motor system is an important and very complex component of the nervous system. It is responsible for controlling all volitional movements.
- The motor system is composed of many parts, including the primary and association cortex, the basal ganglia, the cerebellum, the thalamus, the pyramidal and extrapyramidal tracts, and the neuromuscular junction. Either directly or indirectly, all of these components of the motor system communicate with each other through highly complex pathways within the nervous system.
- Damage at any level of the motor system can result in a movement disorder. When the damage affects the muscles of speech production, the result can be a motor speech disorder.

STUDY QUESTIONS

1. What is the cerebral cortex, and why is it important?
2. What are cranial nerve nuclei, and where are they located?
3. Describe the difference between tracts and nerves.
4. Describe the association cortex and its importance in formulating a movement.

5. How are the functions of the primary cortex different from the functions of the association cortex?
6. What roles do the basal ganglia and cerebellum play in the creation of a movement?
7. How is it known that movements do not originate in the primary motor cortex?
8. What is the difference between the pyramidal and extrapyramidal tracts?
9. Describe the anatomical distinction between lower and upper motor neurons.
10. What happens at the neuromuscular junction?

CHAPTER

4

Flaccid Dysarthria

(continued)

Each of the next seven chapters of this textbook examines one motor speech disorder. They discuss the neurological basis for the disorder, the most common etiologies, the various speech characteristics, and the available treatment options. This chapter examines flaccid dysarthria, a dysarthria associated with damage to lower motor neurons. Chapters 5 and 6 cover spastic dysarthria and unilateral upper motor neuron dysarthria, respectively. Both of these dysarthrias are identified with upper motor neuron damage. Chapters 7, 8, and 9 will discuss ataxic, hypokinetic, and hyperkinetic dysarthria, respectively. These three dysarthrias are associated with damage to some of the most complex areas of the brain. Ataxic dysarthria is caused by damage to the cerebellum. Hypokinetic and hyperkinetic dysarthria both result from damage to the basal ganglia. Chapter 10 examines mixed dysarthria, which is caused by damage to multiple areas of the nervous system. Chapter 11, the last chapter, discusses apraxia of speech. Although not a dysarthria, apraxia of speech is classified as a motor speech disorder. It is most often associated with damage to the left frontal lobe of the brain. So, with that as an introduction to the remainder of the book, the discussion of flaccid dysarthria can begin.

DEFINITIONS OF FLACCID DYSARTHRIA

Most published definitions of flaccid dysarthria emphasize at least two specific characteristics of this disorder. First, they mention that flaccid dysarthria is caused by impairments of the lower motor neurons in the cranial or spinal nerves. This is important, because it indicates that this dysarthria is the result of damage to the peripheral nervous system. Second, most definitions include a statement that individuals with flaccid dysarthria have weakness in the speech or respiratory musculature and that this weakness results in the distinctive qualities of this motor speech disorder. The following two definitions by Darley et al. and Dworkin highlight some of the major characteristics of flaccid dysarthria.

> Damage to lower motor neurons that innervate the respiratory musculature or to the cranial nerves that innervate the speech musculature results in speech changes collectively designated *flaccid dysarthria*. The specific acoustic features depend upon which nerves are affected and the relative degree of weakness that results from damage to them. (Darley et al., 1975, pp. 109–110)

> Patients with [flaccid] dysarthria almost always present with slow-labored articulation, marked degrees of hypernasal resonance, and hoarse-breathy phonation. These characteristics are caused by paralysis, weakness, hypotonicity, atrophy, and hypoactive reflexes of involved speech subsystem musculature owing to damage to their cranial nerve supply or to inherent muscular disease. (Dworkin, 1991, p. 13)

NEUROLOGICAL BASIS OF FLACCID DYSARTHRIA

As was just mentioned, flaccid dysarthria is caused by damage to motor neurons of the PNS. These motor neurons are commonly known by two different names. They sometimes are called *lower motor neurons* because they are part of the PNS. The term *lower* distinguishes these motor neurons of the PNS from the motor neurons of the CNS, which are called *upper* motor neurons. Figure 4–1 illustrates the relationship between lower and upper motor neurons. These motor neurons also are known sometimes as the *final common pathway* because they are the last and only "road" that the neural impulses from the upper motor neurons can travel along to reach the muscles. Flaccid dysarthria can be caused by any disorder that disrupts the flow of neural impulses along the lower motor neurons that innervate the muscles of respiration, phonation, articulation, prosody, or resonance.

Cranial Nerves of Speech Production

There are six pairs of cranial nerves that play a vital role in speech production: trigeminal, facial, glossopharyngeal, vagus, accessory, and hypoglossal. These six nerves are sometimes called the *cranial nerves of speech production*. They are important because the lower motor neurons

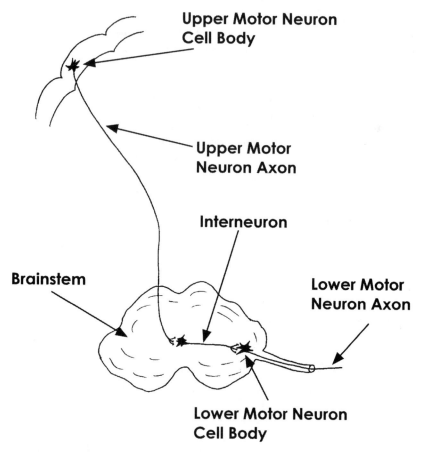

Figure 4–1. Upper motor neurons transmit motor impulses within the central nervous system and ultimately send these impulses to the lower motor neurons in the cranial or spinal nerves.

inside these nerves transmit motor impulses from the upper motor neurons to the muscles used in speech production. Normal speech production requires that these cranial nerves transmit their motor impulses accurately. If a cranial nerve is somehow damaged, the motor impulses it sends to the muscles are likely to be distorted or perhaps even stopped completely. In either case, the damage to the cranial nerve will affect the accurate production of speech.

Many different processes can harm these cranial nerves used in speech production. For example, a brainstem stroke can injure a cranial nerve by disrupting the flow of blood to the cell bodies of its lower motor neurons. Likewise, a growing tumor can compress a cranial nerve to such a degree that its function is compromised. Viral or bacterial infections can damage the tissue of the nerve directly. Physical trauma can damage a cranial nerve, such as when a fractured bone compresses or cuts the nerve. Surgical accidents also might cause damage, in that the slip of a scalpel can nick or completely sever one of these nerves.

If any of these conditions involve the cranial nerves of speech production, the result can be flaccid dysarthria. However, not all injuries to these cranial nerves cause every characteristic of flaccid dysarthria. The specific characteristics of this dysarthria depend on which nerve or combination of nerves is damaged. For example, damage to a branch of the vagus nerve can cause hypernasal speech, one of the most common characteristics of flaccid dysarthria. On the other hand, damage to the hypoglossal nerve can cause distorted productions of lingual consonants, another common characteristic of this dysarthria. If both the vagus and hypoglossal nerves are damaged, the result can be speech that is hypernasal *and* has distorted consonants. Accordingly, the following sections of this chapter examine each of the six cranial nerves involved in speech production, with particular emphasis placed on the consequences of injury to these nerves.

Trigeminal Nerve (V)

The trigeminal nerve is attached to the brainstem at the level of the pons. As it courses out from the brainstem, it divides into three main branches: ophthalmic, maxillary, and mandibular (see Figure 4–2). The most important of these for speech production is the mandibular branch. It innervates the masseter, pterygoid, mylohyoid, and other mandibular muscles that elevate and lower the jaw. It also innervates the tensor veli palatini muscle in the velum, which helps elevate the velum.

Unilateral damage to the trigeminal nerve can result in weakness or paralysis in the jaw and velar muscles that are on the same side as the damage. In such cases, an individual's jaw might deviate toward the affected side when it is opened. Over time, the gradual loss of tissue in the affected jaw muscle (muscular atrophy) may cause a slightly asymmetrical facial appearance. Fortunately, unilateral damage to the trigeminal nerve seldom affects speech production significantly because the jaw and velar muscles on the unaffected side of the body are usually strong enough to compensate for the weakened muscles on the affected side.

However, bilateral damage to the trigeminal nerve can have a very serious effect on articulation. (*Bilateral damage* means that the trigemi-

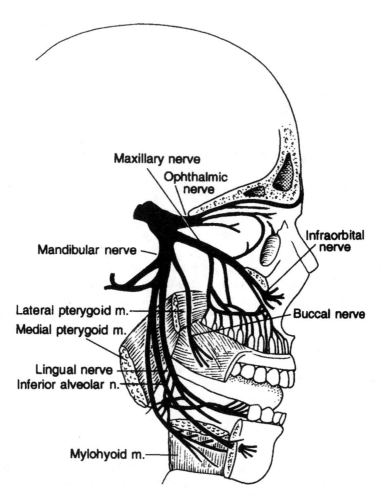

Figure 4–2. The trigeminal nerve has three main branches: ophthalmic, maxillary, and mandibular. (From *Anatomy and Physiology for Speech, Language, and Hearing* [p. 434], by J. Seikel, D. King, and D. Drumright, 1997, San Diego: Singular Publishing Group, Inc. Copyright 1997 by Singular Publishing Group, Inc. Reprinted with permission.)

nal nerve branching out from the left side of the brainstem *and* the one branching out from the right side of the brainstem have both been injured or impaired.) If the bilateral damage is severe, affected individuals cannot raise their jaw sufficiently to produce most consonant and vowel phonemes, especially those requiring bilabial, linguadental, or linguapalatal contact. Furthermore, their rate of speech is often slowed by this reduced ability to elevate the jaw. Hypernasality also may occur after bilateral damage to this nerve because of its innervation of the tensor veli palatini muscle.

Facial Nerve (VII)

The facial cranial nerve branches out from the brainstem just below the trigeminal nerve (see Figure 4–3). As it courses to the muscles of the face, it divides into two major branches. For the most part, the cervicofacial branch innervates the muscles of the lower face through its buccal, lingual, and mandibular subbranches. The temporofacial branch innervates the muscles of the upper face through its temporal and

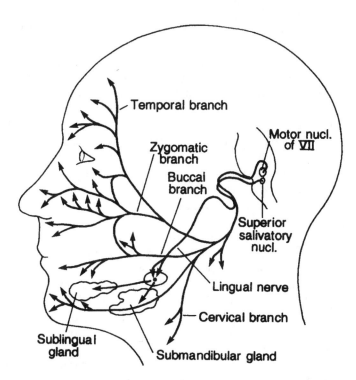

Figure 4–3. The major branches of the facial nerve (VII). (From *Anatomy and Physiology for Speech, Language, and Hearing* [p. 438], by J. Seikel, D. King, and D. Drumright, 1997, San Diego: Singular Publishing Group, Inc. Copyright 1997 by Singular Publishing Group, Inc. Reprinted with permission.)

zygomatic subbranches. Damage to the facial nerve can affect the muscles of the entire face on the same (ipsilateral) side as the lesion if it occurs above the point where the facial nerve divides into its cervicofacial and temporofacial branches. In such cases, all the muscles on the same side of the face as the damage will demonstrate some degree of weakness or paralysis. The result of this facial nerve damage will likely be a facial droop of the eyelid, mouth, cheek, and other structures on the affected side of the face. If the facial nerve damage occurs to just one of these branches, only the muscles innervated by that branch will be affected. For example, if the damage affects the cervicofacial branch, the muscles of the lips will be affected, and the production of bilabial or labiodental sounds may be distorted.

Upper Motor Neuron Innervation of the Facial Nerve

There is a difference in how the upper motor neurons of the corticobulbar tract innervate the lower motor neurons in the two branches of the facial nerve (see Figure 4–4). The branch of the facial nerve that serves the upper face receives *bilateral* upper motor neuron innervation from both the right and left corticobulbar tracts. This means, for example, that unilateral damage to the right corticobulbar tract will not result in weakness or paralysis in the upper part of the left side of the face because the left corticobulbar tract also innervates this branch of the facial nerve. As a result, the upper face will still receive some upper motor neuron innervation despite the damage to the right corticobulbar tract. Consequently, there will be fairly normal contractions of all the muscles in the upper part of the face on both sides.

Upper motor neuron innervation is different, however, for the branch of the facial nerve serving the muscles of the lower face. This branch of the facial nerve only receives unilateral upper motor neuron innervation from the opposite (contralateral) side of the brain. Because of this unilateral innervation, right corticobulbar tract damage will result in weakness or paralysis on the left side of the lower face. Conversely, left corticobulbar tract damage will result in weakness or paralysis on the right side of the lower face

In summary, unilateral upper motor neuron damage in one cerebral hemisphere will result in nearly normal upper face movements of the eyebrow, forehead, and eyelids on both sides of the face. However, movements of the cheek and mouth on the side of the face that is opposite to the site of lesion will be notably weak, and these two parts of the lower face will probably have reduced range of motion. The type of

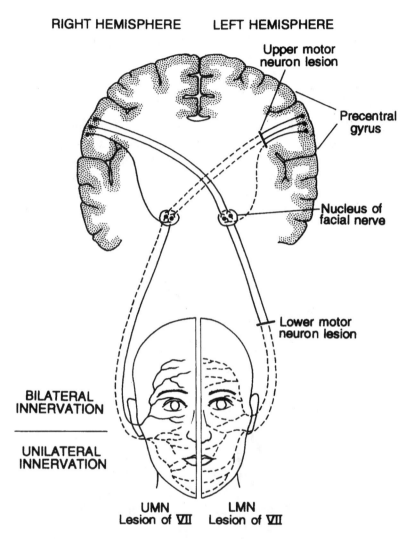

Figure 4–4. A unilateral lesion to the upper motor neurons that inner-vate the facial nerve only will affect the muscles of the lower face. This is because that branch of the facial nerve receives only unilateral upper motor neuron innervation. In contrast, the branch of the facial nerve serving the upper face receives bilateral upper motor neuron innerva-tion. Lower motor neuron lesions will affect all muscles below the point of damage. (From *Anatomy and Physiology for Speech, Language, and Hearing* [p. 436], by J. Seikel, D. King, and D. Drumright, 1997, San Diego: Singular Publishing Group, Inc. Copyright 1997 by Singular Publishing Group, Inc. Reprinted with permission.)

dysarthria that can result from unilateral upper motor neuron damage is known, not surprisingly, as unilateral upper motor neuron dysarthria. It is discussed in Chapter 6.

Glossopharyngeal Nerve (IX)

This cranial nerve originates in the brainstem at the medulla (see Figure 4–5). It courses out to the pharynx where it innervates the stylopharyngeus and superior pharyngeal constrictor muscles. These muscles assist in the elevation and opening of the upper pharynx. Eliciting the gag reflex

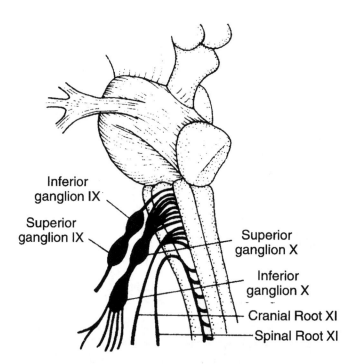

Figure 4–5. The glossopharyngeal nerve (IX) branches off from the brainstem just above the vagus nerve (X) and courses to the pharynx and tongue. (From *Anatomy and Physiology for Speech, Language, and Hearing* [p. 442], by J. Seikel, D. King, and D. Drumright, 1997, San Diego: Singular Publishing Group, Inc. Copyright 1997 by Singular Publishing Group, Inc. Reprinted with permission.)

is one way to assess the function of this cranial nerve. The full importance of the glossopharyngeal nerve on speech is difficult to determine because damage to it also usually will affect the vagus nerve, a cranial nerve that definitely makes significant contributions to speech production. Nevertheless, the glossopharyngeal nerve probably plays a role in speech resonance and phonation by shaping the pharynx into the appropriate positions needed to produce various phonemes correctly.

Vagus Nerve (X)

The vagus nerve is one of the most important cranial nerves for speech production (see Figure 4–6). Its place of origin is in the brainstem at the medulla, just below the glossopharyngeal cranial nerve. It courses out from the medulla in close proximity to the glossopharyngeal and accessory cranial nerves. The vagus nerve is very long and has many branches serving such varied parts of the body as the larynx, intestines, heart, and velum, to name but a few. Three branches of the vagus nerve have special importance for motor speech production: the pharyngeal branch, the external superior laryngeal nerve branch, and the recurrent nerve branch.

Pharyngeal Branch

The pharyngeal branch of the vagus nerve provides motor innervation for many muscles of the pharynx, including the musculus uvulae, levator veli palatini, salpingopharyngeus, palatopharyngeus, and the superior and middle pharyngeal constrictor muscles. Damage to the pharyngeal branch of the vagus nerve can affect the movement of the velum. For instance, unilateral damage to this branch can result in the affected side of the velum hanging visibly lower than the other side. In most cases, unilateral damage usually does not result in hypernasal speech because the velar muscles on the unaffected side usually will be able to raise the velum sufficiently to ensure adequate velopharyngeal closure on nonnasal phonemes.

However, bilateral damage to the pharyngeal branch of the vagus nerve can have a very significant effect on resonance. (Remember, *bilateral damage* means that both the left and right branches of a nerve have been injured in some manner.) When the damage is bilateral, nearly all the muscles of the velum will demonstrate weakness or paralysis. The result will be speech with moderate to severe hypernasality. In addition, the pressure consonants (stops, fricatives, and affricates) may be weak and distorted because of the nasal emission of air through the unsealed velopharyngeal port.

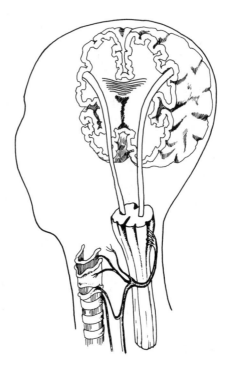

Figure 4–6. The many branches of the vagus nerve are very complex and serve many parts of the body. This drawing shows the vagus nerve branching from the brainstem and coursing to the larynx, velum, and pharynx.

External Superior Laryngeal Nerve Branch

The external superior laryngeal branch of the vagus nerve innervates the cricothyroid muscle of the larynx. This muscle helps to stretch and tense the vocal folds during speech. As a consequence, this muscle is essential in controlling vocal pitch. Unilateral damage to this nerve branch usually results in only modest difficulty in varying pitch. However, bilateral damage can cause significant problems. When the damage is bilateral, the cricothyroid muscle's ability to stretch and tense the vocal folds is greatly reduced. In such cases, an affected individual's voice may exhibit decreased loudness, increased breathiness, and notable difficulty in changing vocal pitch.

Recurrent Nerve Branch

This branch of the vagus nerve gets its name from the "double-back" route it takes as it travels from the brainstem to the larynx. The fibers of the recurrent nerve branch off from the vagus nerve after it leaves the cranium and course down near the heart before turning upward. They then travel upward along the trachea until finally reaching the larynx. The recurrent nerve supplies the motor innervation to all the intrinsic muscles of the larynx, except the cricothyroid muscle, which is inner-vated by the external superior laryngeal nerve. The recurrent nerve is a vital contributor to phonation, because it supplies the motor innerva-tion for all the adductor and abductor muscles of the vocal folds.

Unilateral damage to the recurrent nerve will cause the vocal fold on the affected side to be fixed in the paramedian position, which means that the fold is halfway between being fully adducted or abducted. An individual with unilateral vocal fold paralysis will demonstrate a breathy phonation and have decreased vocal loudness. Bilateral damage to the recurrent nerve can fix both vocal folds in the paramedian posi-tion. When both vocal folds are in this position, they will probably still be close enough together to permit phonation on exhalation. However, this phonation will be very breathy and hoarse. Phonation on inhalation (inhalatory stridor) also might be evident because the vocal folds are fixed in this position during inhalation as well as exhalation.

Accessory Nerve (XI)

The accessory nerve is unique in that it is not a "pure" cranial nerve. It also contains neurons that branch out from the spinal cord. The cranial neurons of this nerve originate in the medulla just below the vagus nerve (see Figure 4–7). In fact, many of its motor neuron axons merge with the vagus nerve shortly after they leave the medulla. These cra-nial motor neurons from the accessory nerve, working in conjunction with the vagus nerve, help innervate the intrinsic muscles of the velum, pharynx, and larynx. The spinal components of the accessory nerve supply motor innervation for the sternocleidomastoid and trapezius muscles. Because the neurons of this cranial nerve are so closely inte-grated with those of the vagus nerve, it is practically impossible to sep-arate the functions of the two. Suffice it to say that damage to the cra-nial components of the accessory nerve almost always will affect the vagus nerve as well and vice versa.

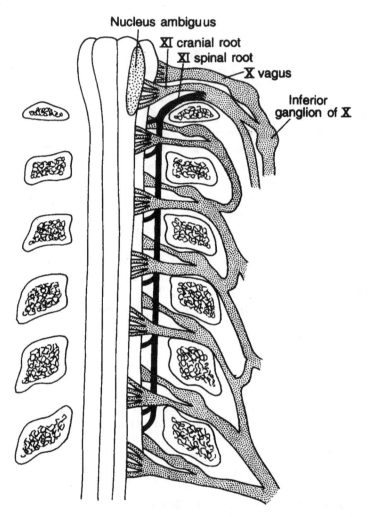

Figure 4–7. The cranial root and spinal roots of the accessory nerve (XI). (From *Anatomy and Physiology for Speech, Language, and Hearing* [p. 446], by J. Seikel, D. King, and D. Drumright, 1997, San Diego: Singular Publishing Group, Inc. Copyright 1997 by Singular Publishing Group, Inc. Reprinted with permission.)

Hypoglossal Nerve (XII)

The hypoglossal cranial nerve originates in the medulla and courses to the tongue. This cranial nerve provides the motor innervation for all the intrinsic and most of the extrinsic muscles of the tongue. Unilateral damage to the hypoglossal cranial nerve results in weakness or paralysis in the half of the tongue that is on the same side as the nerve damage. If the damage is severe enough, the tongue muscles on the damaged side will eventually atrophy, leaving that half of the tongue shrunken. Furthermore, when the tongue is protruded, it will deviate toward the affected side, because only half of the posterior genioglossus muscle is being contracted. Bilateral damage to the hypoglossal nerve will result in an overall weakness of the tongue. The range of tongue movement also will be reduced. Muscle atrophy will occur on both sides of the tongue in cases of bilateral damage to the hypoglossal nerve.

As with the branch of the facial nerve that innervates the lower face, the hypoglossal cranial nerve primarily receives unilateral innervation from the upper motor neurons. This means, for example, that most of the innervation for the right hypoglossal nerve comes only from the upper motor neurons of the corticobulbar tract that are in the left hemisphere of the brain. Damage to those left upper motor neurons will result in weakness in the right side of the tongue. Conversely, damage to the right upper motor neurons will result in weakness in the left side of the tongue.

Imprecise articulation is the primary characteristic of an individual with hypoglossal nerve damage. In cases of unilateral damage, the articulatory distortion will probably be mild, because the unaffected side of the tongue can usually compensate for the weakened movements of the affected side. Bilateral damage, however, can have a much more significant effect on articulation. In these cases, phonemes requiring elevation of the tip or back of the tongue will be produced with notable distortion (Duffy, 1995). Slow lingual movements also will be evident.

Spinal Nerves

The spinal nerves originate along the length of the spinal cord, from the cervical and thoracic sections down to the lumbar region. Many of the spinal nerves serve an important role in motor speech production because they provide the motor innervation for the muscles of respiration. One of the most important nerves of respiration is the phrenic nerve. It is a spinal nerve that originates from the cervical section of the spinal cord and provides the motor innervation of the diaphragm. The other muscles of inhalation and exhalation are innervated by the spinal nerves that originate along the cervical and thoracic portions of the spinal cord.

Damage to the cervical and thoracic spinal nerves can affect respiration and, thereby, can affect speech. In most instances, however, the damage must be quite widespread before a significant impairment of respiration will be evident. An exception to this is damage to the phrenic nerve. Damage to this nerve can paralyze the diaphragm and result in significantly weakened inhalation. Individuals with impaired respiratory abilities may demonstrate decreased speech loudness as a result of reduced subglottic air pressure. Furthermore, these individuals may demonstrate shortened speech phrasing because of the reduced amount of air available for phonation. This shortened phrasing would almost certainly affect the prosody of their speech as well. Individuals with impaired respiration also may attempt to speak in longer phrases than their air supply will allow, resulting in a breathy or strained vocal quality towards the end of an utterance (known as "speaking on residual air").

ETIOLOGIES OF FLACCID DYSARTHRIA

Flaccid dysarthria can be caused by anything that disrupts the flow of motor impulses along the cranial or spinal nerves that innervate the muscles of speech production. Several conditions that damage lower motor neurons were briefly mentioned earlier in this chapter, such as brainstem stroke, tumors, and so forth. In the following paragraphs, the conditions that can cause flaccid dysarthria are examined in more detail.

Physical Trauma

Surgical trauma, head injury, and neck injury are common etiologies of flaccid dysarthria. Duffy (1995) indicated that these injuries caused 34% of flaccid dysarthria cases at the Mayo Clinic during a 21-year period—the highest percentage of all reported causes of this dysarthria. This high occurrence probably should not be surprising, given that physical damage leading to flaccid dysarthria can occur anywhere along the course of lower motor neurons, from the cell bodies in the brainstem to the neuromuscular junction.

Some of the surgical procedures that can lead to inadvertent damage to the cranial nerves of speech production include carotid endarterectomy (the removal of plaque deposits in a carotid artery), cardiac surgery, the removal of head and neck tumors, and dental surgery. In most of these cases, a cranial nerve is cut accidentally because of its nearness to the surgical site. Head and neck trauma resulting from motor vehicle accidents, blows to the head, and falls also can damage the cranial nerves of speech production. Broken bones from this type of trauma can compress or cut one of these cranial nerves. It also is possible that the rotational forces of such trauma can twist or stretch a nerve enough to cause damage. In any of these instances, the cranial nerve will be impaired in its ability to carry motor impulses, resulting in weakness or paralysis in the muscles innervated by the nerve.

Brainstem Stroke

Flaccid dysarthria can be caused by a stroke, which is more frequently called a *cerebrovascular accident* (CVA) by medical professionals. A stroke occurs when the blood flow to the brain is interrupted because an artery breaks or is blocked. In either case, brain tissue is damaged from the lack of blood flow and the disruption of the neurons' metabolic processes. As with all other parts of the brain, the brainstem is rich with arterial blood flow, and when a stroke occurs in one of the brainstem arteries, the neurons served by that artery can be destroyed.

A brainstem stroke can directly affect the cranial nerves, because the cell bodies of lower motor neurons (the cranial nerve nuclei) are located within the brainstem. When the blood supply to these cell bodies is blocked, many of the neurons will eventually die. Naturally, this will impair the ability of the cranial nerves to transmit motor impulses to the muscles. The degree of impairment depends on the number of lower motor neurons that are lost to a stroke. If only a few neurons are affected, the resulting impairment of motor innervation might be minimal. If many of a cranial nerve's motor neurons are affected, numerous muscles innervated by that cranial nerve will be weakened or paralyzed.

It also is very possible for a single brainstem stroke to damage more than one cranial nerve. If the stroke is large enough to damage the cells in more than one cranial nerve nuclei, it will affect more than one cranial nerve. In fact, the damaging stroke does not have to be all that massive before it will affect more than one cranial nerve. Many cranial nerve nuclei are in close proximity in the brainstem. For example, the cranial nerve nuclei of the glossopharyngeal, vagus, and accessory nerves are quite close to each other in the brainstem. A single brainstem stroke in that area may very well affect the lower motor neurons in all three of those cranial nerves.

Myasthenia Gravis

Myasthenia gravis is a disease that affects the neuromuscular junction, which is the point where lower motor neurons meet muscle tissue. The primary symptom of this disease is the rapid fatigue of muscular contractions over a short period of time, with recovery occurring after rest. Myasthenia gravis is caused by antibodies that damage the parts of muscle tissue that receive the neurotransmitter acetylcholine from the lower motor neurons. It is the reception of acetylcholine at the muscle that triggers a muscular contraction. With the loss of too many acetylcholine receptors, the muscle is not able to use all of the acetylcholine being produced by the motor neuron. Consequently, the muscle cannot maintain the strength of its contractions over time. The result is rapid fatigue and weakness. With rest, however, the muscle can again make more efficient use of the acetylcholine, and stronger contractions will occur once again. A very temporary treatment for this disorder is an injection of edrophonium chloride (Tensilon), which can almost immediately improve muscle contractions for several minutes. After a brief period, however, the strength of the muscular contractions rapidly deteriorates again.

The speech characteristics of individuals with myasthenia gravis include hypernasality, decreased loudness, breathy voice quality, and decreased articulatory imprecision during prolonged speaking tasks. In motor speech evaluations, a stress test is often included to help determine the presence of this disease. Usually, this test requires the patient to count from 1 to 100 or to read a lengthy paragraph.

Guillain-Barré Syndrome

Guillain-Barré syndrome results in the progressive inflammatory loss of the myelin sheath around axons (demyelination). The exact cause of this disorder is undetermined, but it frequently occurs after certain kinds of infections and immunizations. The demyelination usually occurs in the PNS and tends to affect motor neurons more than sensory neurons. The progression of this disorder is usually quite rapid, often developing over a period of days or a few weeks. This is in striking contrast to some of the better-known progressive neurological disorders such as Parkinson disease, which typically progress over a period of months or years.

In severe cases, Guillain-Barré syndrome can result in a near total paralysis of the entire body. Complaints of weakness and numbness in the limbs are common early symptoms of this disorder. Other early symptoms include flaccid dysarthria and dysphagia, once the demyelination affects the cranial nerves. Recovery from Guillain-Barré syndrome is usually good, but about 5% of affected individuals die during the acute stages of the disorder (Warlow, 1991). The typical recovery occurs over a period of weeks or months. Persons with the most severe cases, however, might not fully recover and may always have some permanent weakness.

Polio

Polio is an infectious viral disease that attacks the cell bodies of lower motor neurons. Although vaccines have reduced the incidence of this disease greatly, unvaccinated individuals can become infected after close contact with a recently vaccinated child (Wiederholt, 1995). Polio most frequently affects the cervical and thoracic spinal nerves, which often results in isolated respiratory weakness. When there is respiratory weakness, the motor speech symptoms can include labored inhalation during speech, shortened speech phrases, speaking on residual air, and decreased loudness. Unfortunately, a polio infection is not always restricted to the spinal nerves. It also can affect the cranial nerves. In about 10 to 15% of polio cases, the virus can damage the lower motor neurons in the trigeminal, facial, glossopharyngeal, and vagus nerves (Duffy, 1995), resulting in weakness in the muscles innervated by those nerves.

Other Causes of Flaccid Dysarthria

Although there are many additional disorders that can cause flaccid dysarthria, a short summary of a just few follows. **Tumors** growing in or near the brainstem can compromise a cranial nerve's ability to transmit its neural impulses to muscles. Tumors occurring along the course of a cranial nerve's pathway, such as in the neck or in any orofacial structure, also can affect the nerve's functioning. **Muscular dystrophy** is a disease that causes a progressive degeneration of muscle tissue. It can result in weakness in many muscles served by the cranial nerves, such as the tongue, face, and pharynx. **Progressive bulbar palsy** is a disorder that can affect both upper and lower motor neurons, although it often is present only in the lower motor neurons. When the lower motor neurons are affected, progressive bulbar palsy can cause flaccid dysarthria. When it is present in both sets of motor neurons, it can result in a mixed dysarthria, usually of the flaccid-spastic type (see Chapter 10).

SPEECH CHARACTERISTICS OF FLACCID DYSARTHRIA

The following section of this chapter discusses the typical speech characteristics of flaccid dysarthria. The effects of flaccid dysarthria on resonance, articulation, phonation, respiration, and prosody are discussed. It is important to remember, however, that not all individuals with flaccid dysarthria will demonstrate deficits in each of these areas, although some will. Furthermore, the relative severity level within each area will not necessarily be the same for any two patients. Individual variations in motor speech deficits are common for all the dysarthrias, even when the affected individuals share the same type of dysarthria. Because of these variations, it is important to look for clusters of symptoms when trying to diagnose a particular type of dysarthria. Once a cluster of symptoms has been identified, determine which type of dysarthria it most closely represents. This holds true for the diagnosis of any motor speech disorder, not just flaccid dysarthria.

Resonance

In their landmark study of dysarthria, Darley et al. (1969a, 1969b) examined the abnormal speech characteristics of 30 subjects with flaccid dysarthria. Table 4–1 ranks these subjects' nine most prominent speech errors. **Hypernasality** was the most noticeable error. It was present in the speech of 25 of the 30 subjects. Hypernasality is certainly an important diagnostic marker for flaccid dysarthria. Although it is not unique to flaccid dysarthria, it tends to be more noticeable in this type of dysarthria compared to the other dysarthrias. Other resonance related problems in flaccid dysarthria include **nasal emission** due to incom-

Table 4–1. Most Common Speech Production Errors in 30 Individuals With Flaccid Dysarthria

Rank	Speech Production Errors
1	Hypernasality
2	Imprecise consonants
3	Breathiness (continuous)
4	Monopitch
5	Nasal emission
6	Audible inspiration
7	Harsh voice quality
8	Short phrases
9	Monoloudness

Note: From "Clusters of Diagnostic Patterns of Dysarthria," by F. L. Darley, A. E. Aronson, and J. R. Brown; 1969, *Journal of Speech and Hearing Research,* 12, p. 251. Copyright 1969 by American Speech-Language-Hearing Association. Reprinted with permission.

plete velopharyngeal closure, **weak pressure consonants** caused by decreased intraoral air pressure, and **shortened phrases**, which are the result of wasted air that escapes through the nasal cavity during speech. All of these resonance deficits primarily reflect bilateral damage to the pharyngeal branch of the vagus nerve, because it innervates most of the muscles of the velum.

Articulation

Imprecise consonant production was the second most prominent abnormal speech characteristic of flaccid dysarthria reported by Darley et al. (1969a, 1969b). There can be a large range of severity for misarticulated phonemes in individuals with flaccid dysarthria, from only a mild distortion to complete unintelligibility. Damage to the facial and hypoglossal nerves are usually cited as reasons for these problems with the production of consonant phonemes (Duffy, 1995). Bilateral damage to the facial nerve can have a significant effect on the production of bilabial and labiodental phonemes, as well as with consonants and vowels requiring lip rounding. Bilateral damage to the hypoglossal nerve will likely result in misarticulations of phonemes requiring the elevation of the tongue, especially the tongue tip. For example, a damaged hypoglossal nerve can affect the production of the linguadental and linguapalatal phonemes, such as /j/ and /l/. In severe cases of bilateral hypoglossal nerve damage, the production of the linguavelar phonemes also will be impaired.

Damage to the trigeminal nerve also can affect articulation. As was mentioned previously, bilateral damage to this nerve can result in difficulty elevating the jaw sufficiently to bring the articulators into contact with each other. Without proper jaw elevation, it may be impossible for an affected individual to accurately produce any of the consonants and most of the vowels. Such an individual may need to elevate the jaw by hand or use a device known as a jaw sling before intelligible speech is possible. Other treatment options are discussed later in this chapter.

Phonation

Another common abnormal speech characteristic of flaccid dysarthria is **phonatory incompetence** (Darley et al., 1969a, 1969b). This term refers to the incomplete adduction of the vocal folds during phonation. It is caused by damage to the recurrent branch of the vagus nerve, which provides motor innervation to almost all of the intrinsic muscles of the larynx. Injury to this cranial nerve can leave the vocal fold adductor and abductor muscles weak or paralyzed. If the adductor muscles are primarily affected, the vocal folds will not meet with enough strength to produce a clear phonation. The result will be phonation that has a **breathy voice quality**, which can almost sound like a whisper in severe cases. If the abductor muscles are primarily affected, the vocal folds will not be able to fully abduct during inhalation. When abduction is incomplete, there can be an audible inhalation stridor.

As with hypernasality, phonatory incompetence is an especially valuable confirmatory sign for the diagnosis of flaccid dysarthria. It can be quite prominent in cases of flaccid dysarthria to a degree that is not found in the other dysarthrias (Duffy, 1995). Moreover, the combined presence of hypernasality and phonatory incompetence is the strongest confirmatory sign that flaccid dysarthria is the correct diagnosis.

Respiration

Weakened respiration may or may not be a component of flaccid dysarthria. If the cervical and thoracic spinal nerves responsible for innervating the diaphragm and the intercostal muscles are damaged, the result can be decreased inhalation or impaired control of exhalation during speech. In either instance, the affected individuals will not have adequate amounts of subglottic air pressure for speech. Without enough subglottic air, the speech of individuals with flaccid dysarthria may demonstrate **reduced loudness** and **shortened phrase length**. Their speech may have a **strained vocal quality** if they speak on residual air to prolong the length of their phrases. Of course, reduced loudness, shortened phrase length, and strained vocal quality will affect prosody. In addition, Darley et al. (1975) mentioned that individuals with weakened respiration can also demonstrate monoloudness and monopitch.

A Problem of Respiration or Phonation?

Many individuals with flaccid dysarthria inhale frequently during speech, which can adversely affect the prosody of their speech. Although frequent inhalations are usually easy to identify, it is sometimes difficult to determine whether the problem is one of air wastage because of poor laryngeal valving or reduced vital capacity because of weakened respiration. In either case, the affected individual will probably demonstrate reduced loudness, shortened phrase length, and strained vocal quality in conversational speech. But how is a clinician to determine whether the problem is one of respiration or phonation? Duffy (1995) described a simple procedure to help determine which is the most likely cause of this problem.

1. Ask the individual to first produce a good cough and then listen to how "sharp" it sounds. A breathy, feeble cough may indicate weakness in the vocal fold adductor muscles, inadequate respiration, or perhaps both.
2. Then ask the individual to produce a hard glottal stop; again listen to how sharp it sounds. Producing a hard glottal stop requires firm closure of the vocal folds but little respiratory effort. Consequently, the individual who produces a breathy cough *and* a sharp glottal stop may be demonstrating poor

respiration. In turn, a breathy cough and a weak glottal stop might indicate that the cause of the air supply problem is either weak laryngeal closure or a combination of weak laryngeal and respiratory functioning.

Prosody

Individuals with flaccid dysarthria may demonstrate speech that has **monopitch** and **monoloudness**. Darley et al. (1969a, 1969b) noted both of these prosodic errors in their subjects with flaccid dysarthria. It is likely that these qualities are primarily the result of weakened laryngeal muscles that are unable to make the many fine vocal fold adjustments needed for normal pitch and loudness variations. For example, if the cricothyroid muscle is weakened by damage to the superior laryngeal branch of the vagus nerve, it may not be able to tense and stretch the vocal folds sufficiently for normal changes in pitch and loudness. Incidentally, monopitch and monoloudness are not unique to flaccid dysarthria. These two prosodic errors can appear in a number of other dysarthrias, such as spastic and ataxic dysarthria. Consequently, the presence of monopitch and monoloudness are not definite diagnostic markers for flaccid dysarthria, unlike the co-occurrence of hypernasality and phonatory insufficiency.

KEY EVALUATION TASKS
FOR FLACCID DYSARTHRIA

Several evaluation tasks are especially effective in detecting the most notable speech characteristics of flaccid dysarthria. A patient's performance on these tasks should be observed carefully if flaccid dysarthria is suspected.

1. Conversational speech and reading can evoke the errors of resonance (hypernasality), articulation (imprecise consonants), respiration (shortened phrase length), and prosody (monopitch, monoloudness).
2. The alternate motion rate (AMR) task will highlight a slowed rate of phoneme production.
3. A prolonged vowel will be helpful in eliciting the breathy voice quality heard in phonatory incompetence. It also may be useful for observing respiratory weakness.

4. A speech stress test is necessary in suspected cases of myasthenia gravis.

TREATMENT OF FLACCID DYSARTHRIA

The final section of each remaining chapter contains treatment ideas for one of the dysarthrias. Clinicians should know that these sections cover the most practical treatment tasks based on the author's experience; however, they are not exhaustive. No book of this kind can include every treatment idea for such a complex collection of disorders as dysarthria and apraxia of speech. There are additional treatment ideas in other textbooks and research articles. Clinicians are encouraged to search out other treatment options. Three textbooks in particular are recommended for their treatment ideas, as well as for their general examination of motor speech disorders:

- *Motor Speech Disorders: Substrates, Differential Diagnosis, and Management* (Duffy, 1995)
- *Motor Speech Disorders: A Treatment Guide* (Dworkin, 1991)
- *The Source for Dysarthria* (Swigert, 1997)

As has been mentioned several times in this chapter, flaccid dysarthria is caused by damage to the lower motor neurons in six specific cranial nerves. The following treatment options for flaccid dysarthria are grouped according to which cranial nerve is damaged. Of course, flaccid dysarthria is often the result of damage to more than one cranial nerve, so combinations of various treatments are appropriate in those cases. The recommended number of trials in these treatments is only a rough guideline. The needs of patients vary greatly. Some will not be able to complete the recommended trials; others may benefit from more than the recommended trials. Clinicians will need to adjust the treatment tasks according to the requirements and abilities of their patients.

Before examining the specific treatment tasks, a few words should be said about oral strengthening exercises. Because muscular weakness is such a common characteristic of flaccid dysarthria, many clinicians assume that strengthening tasks should be an important part of a treatment plan. However, the value of these activities as a treatment for flaccid dysarthria is open to question. To date there are no definitive research studies that have shown that these exercises make significant contributions to the recovery of speech production. Duffy (1995) made one of the strongest points against strengthening exercises when he said, "That strengthening exercise may be unnecessary is supported by the facts that the tongue and lips use only 10% to 30% of their maximum forces for speech, and the jaw only 2%, and that up to one third of motor nerve fibers can be lost before functional impairments are encountered" (p. 398).

Nevertheless, these types of exercises are recommended (with qualifications) by a number of writers (Dworkin, 1991; Linebaugh, 1983). Swigert (1997) suggested that strengthening exercises are most often appropriate for patients who have either a severe weakness in the articulators or only a mild weakness. According to Swigert, patients whose flaccid dysarthria is so severe that it prevents most attempts at articulation may show improvement with strengthening exercises. On the other hand, patients with only a very mild weakness may benefit from a course of strengthening exercises that they can perform on their own and at their own pace. Swigert's suggestion appears to be an appropriate course of action until clinical studies have settled the question of whether strengthening tasks are an effective treatment for flaccid dysarthria.

Damage to the Trigeminal Cranial Nerve (V)

Unilateral damage to this cranial nerve typically has a negligible effect on speech production. Patients with this type of injury probably will not need significant amounts of treatment. However, bilateral damage to the trigeminal nerve can leave the jaw muscles very weak or, in severe cases, cause an inability to close the jaw. Treatment for bilateral trigeminal nerve damage is designed to strengthen the jaw muscles or to compensate for their weakness.

Jaw Muscle Strengthening

The initial steps in strengthening the jaw muscles should concentrate on merely opening and closing the mouth fully. For example, the patient should attempt to complete 3 sets of 10 full mouth openings and closings each session. Once the patient is able to fully close the mouth, treatment should emphasize increasing the strength of the closure. Dworkin (1991) recommended having the patient bite down on a resistance wedge constructed from tongue blades (Figure 4–8). By

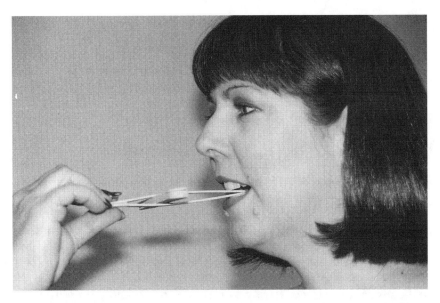

Figure 4–8. A resistance wedge can be used to build jaw strength. (From Dworkin, 1991).

increasing the number of blades in the wedge (from 1 to 5), increasing amounts of jaw muscle strength are needed to bite down completely on the blades. The patients are encouraged to sustain a bite for about 5 seconds on each trial.

A more "hands on" jaw-strengthening exercise employs the clinician's hands to provide resistance to the movement of the patient's jaw. For example, the patient is asked to close the mouth while the clinician firmly holds the chin. Conversely, the patient is asked to open the mouth while the clinician presses upward on the jaw.

Jaw Sling

When the bilateral damage to this cranial nerve is so severe that strengthening exercises are not possible, a jaw sling may be an appropriate treatment option. A jaw sling is a prosthetic device that supports the jaw and lifts it close to the maxilla. By adjusting the amount of supportive jaw elevation provided by the sling, appropriate articulatory contact can be provided for the lower lip and the tongue.

Damage to the Facial Cranial Nerve (VII)

Damage to the facial nerve affects speech production primarily by decreasing lip strength and range of movement. This weakness and reduced range of lip motion results in distorted bilabial and labiodental phonemes. Numerous lip-strengthening exercises are mentioned in the treatment literature.

Lip Strengthening Exercises Using Button and String

Dworkin (1991) described a lip-strengthening task that uses a button and string (Figure 4–9). For this exercise, a nickel-sized button and a 12-inch piece of string are needed. Thread the string through the buttonholes and tie a knot in the end. Place the button against the central incisors and behind the midline of the lips. Instruct the patient to close the lips around the button and resist efforts to pull the button from the mouth. The clinician should rest the middle, ring, and little fingers against the patient's chin and tug the string by the index finger and thumb. The clinician should maintain a steady tugging force that challenges the patient but does not break the lip seal easily. Right or left lip strength can be exercised by placing the button against the teeth and behind the lips at each corner of the mouth. The clinician should pull gently and encourage the patient to press the lips together as tightly as possible for about 5 seconds. Repeat until 10 consecutive trials are completed.

Lip Puckering

In this strengthening task, the patient is asked to pucker the lips fully and hold them in that position for a given amount of time, perhaps 10 seconds. The clinician should determine if the patient is able to move the pucker to one side of the mouth, hold it, and then move it to the other side. Repeat this side-to-side lip puckering movement until 10 consecutive trials are completed.

Holding a Smile

Ask the patient to smile as widely as possible and hold the lips in that position for about 5 to 10 seconds. Swigert (1997) suggested that the clinician use the thumb and index finger to try pushing the lips into a pucker while the patient resists the action by maintaining the smile.

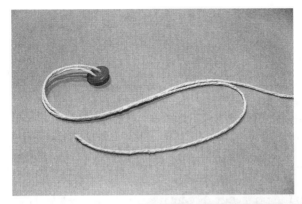

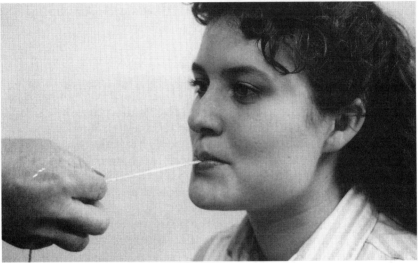

Figure 4–9. Lip strength may be increased by pulling on a button that is placed just behind the lips. (From Dworkin, 1991).

Damage to the Vagus Cranial Nerve (X)

As mentioned previously, damage to the vagus nerve also usually affects the glossopharyngeal and accessory cranial nerves, because all three of these cranial nerves branch out from the brainstem in very close proximity to each other. Moreover, it is often difficult to separate the functions of these cranial nerves because they innervate many of the same anatomical structures. Consequently, it is appropriate to assume that the tasks presented in this section also are suitable treatments for damage to the glossopharyngeal and accessory nerves.

Treatments for Resonance Deficits

Injury to the pharyngeal branch of the vagus nerve can result in weak, incomplete elevation of the velum, which may cause hypernasal resonance. The severity of the hypernasality depends partly on whether the damage to this nerve branch is unilateral or bilateral. Unilateral damage may result in only mild hypernasality, because the unaffected pharyngeal nerve branch from the contralateral side continues to innervate the muscles on the other side of the soft palate. However, bilateral damage to the pharyngeal branch of the vagus nerve usually results in moderate to severe hypernasality, because the muscles on both sides of the soft palate are either weakened or paralyzed.

Surgical and Prosthetic Treatments

Two procedures are used in the surgical treatment of velopharyngeal incompetence. The first is a pharyngeal flap. In this procedure, a flap of tissue from the pharynx is surgically attached to the velum. As a result, much of the velopharyngeal port is closed by this attached flap of tissue. However, the sides of the flap are left loose to provide an opening between the oral and nasal cavities, which, of course, is important for nasal breathing and producing nasal speech sounds. The other surgical procedure used to treat hypernasality is the injection of Teflon or similar substance into the pharynx at the point where the soft palate normally makes contact when it is elevated. The Teflon injection creates a bulge at that point on the pharynx and lessens the distance the velum must elevate before velopharyngeal closure is completed.

The effectiveness of these two procedures in individuals with dysarthria has been inconsistent. They have worked well for some patients but not for others. Teflon injections have had especially mixed results. Because of these variable results, a prosthetic treatment called a palatal lift currently is used more widely than either of the surgical treatments. A palatal lift is essentially a dental retainer that has a rear extension that helps push upward on the velum. Because of this upward push, the device can aid in the elevation of the velum during speech. Duffy (1995) indicated that the palatal lift is the most successful treatment of resonance problems in individuals with dysarthria. However, he also mentioned the characteristics of individuals who are the best candidates for this prosthetic device:

- Hypernasality is their most serious speech production deficit.
- Their medical condition is stable and not deteriorating.
- They have enough teeth onto which the lift can be attached.
- They do not have a hyperactive gag reflex or have significant oral spasticity.
- They have the patience and motivation to use the lift.
- They are able to insert and remove the device independently.

Given these criteria, it should be clear that a palatal lift is not appropriate for all patients, but it, nevertheless, is currently the most effective treatment for individuals with severe hypernasal resonance.

Velar Strengthening Exercises

Numerous researchers agree that velar strengthening and stimulation procedures do little to improve velopharyngeal closure in most cases of flaccid dysarthria (Brookshire, 1992; Dworkin & Johns, 1980). Nevertheless, strengthening exercises may be appropriate in fine tuning velopharyngeal closure in a patient with a palatal lift. During the adjustment period that takes place after the initial placement of a palatal lift, various blowing and sucking tasks may be useful in maximizing the effectiveness of a palatal lift during velopharyngeal closure. Dworkin (1991) recommended a series of velar exercises to increase intraoral air pressure that may be effective in improving velar elevation once the palatal lift is in place. These exercises use increasingly difficult blowing activities, which conclude with the patient inflating a small balloon with their own breath.

Modification of Speech

Modification of speech behaviors can minimize the effects of hypernasality in some patients. These modification procedures include the following tasks:

- **Increase loudness**—The perception of hypernasality can sometimes be minimized by having the patient speak more loudly. Louder speech tends to mask the hypernasal resonance in individuals with flaccid dysarthria. Equally important, the louder speech can often increase intelligibility by simply making it easier for a listener to hear what is being spoken. Modeling appropriate loudness levels is a key component of this treatment. Visual feedback on loudness is also helpful for most patients. Such devices as a sound pressure level meter or a Vocalite can give patients a visual cue as to what the desired loudness should be.

- **Reduce rate of speech**—Reducing the rate of speech also can increase intelligibility and lessen the perception of hypernasality in some individuals with flaccid dysarthria. There are numerous activities for reducing rate (see Chapter 8). One that may be appropriate in cases of flaccid dysarthria is the use of finger or hand tapping to set the appropriate speaking rate. In this procedure, the patient speaks one word or syllable for every tap of the clinician's finger or hand. Generally, slowing rate in this manner increases intelligibility because it allows extra time for the articulators to reach their targets, thus resulting in more precise articulation of phonemes. The slower rate may decrease hypernasality because it can give a slow-moving velum extra time to more fully close the velopharyngeal port during connected speech.

- **More open-position mouth during speech**—Exaggerated jaw movements during speech also can lessen the perception of hypernasality. Swigert (1997) recommended a sequence of steps that can increase the patient's ability to maintain a more open mouth while speaking. First, increase the patient's awareness of what is hypernasal speech. This can be accomplished through clinician modeling and by having the patient read sentences that have either many nasal phonemes or no nasal phonemes. Second, while looking in a mirror, have the patient repeat sentences that contain many open vowels. The patient should try to maintain exaggerated jaw movements while repeating the sentences. Third, the clinician can use negative practice to demonstrate the positive effects of an open mouth posture. For example, the patient is instructed to purposefully keep the mouth nearly closed during speech. With the mouth almost closed, the patient's speech should be noticeably more hypernasal compared to when a wide-open posture is used. Instant replays of video- or audiotape recordings may also be useful in helping the patient hear the difference in hypernasality between the open and closed posture speech.

Treatments for Phonation Deficits

Damage to the recurrent branch of the vagus nerve can cause significant problems of phonation, because this branch innervates nearly all the intrinsic muscles of the larynx. Damage to this nerve branch usually results in breathy or harsh vocal quality, as laryngeal muscle weakness or paralysis prevents the vocal folds from fully adducting. There are several treatment tasks that can bring the vocal folds together more completely during phonation and may result in a clearer, more normal vocal quality.

- **Pushing and pulling procedures**—Sometimes described as *effortful closure techniques*, pushing and pulling procedures help the vocal folds adduct by providing an overall increase in muscle contractions in the torso and neck. Given enough time and practice, these procedures might increase muscle strength in the larynx. Examples of these techniques include having a sitting patient push up on the arms of a chair while phonating an open vowel or having the patient pulling up on the edge of a heavy table while prolonging a vowel.
- **Holding breath**—Holding a deep breath of air requires the ability to fully adduct the vocal folds. The tighter the adduction, the better the air will be held in the lungs. Ask the patient to inhale deeply and hold his or her breath. Use a small mirror under the nostrils to detect leaking air. Work to the point where the patient can hold a breath of air for about 15 seconds over 10 consecutive trials. Be sure to give sufficient rest periods between the trials.
- **Hard glottal attack**—Some patients can demonstrate a better quality phonation when they begin an utterance with a hard glottal attack. Dworkin (1991) described a complete exercise for this procedure. The basic steps are to have the patient hold a deep breath, bear down, and attempt to phonate a tight /a/. This tight phonation should be modified into a more normal vocal quality as soon as possible to avoid the negative side effects of consistent hard glottal attacks during speech.
- **Head turning and sideways pressure on the larynx**—When there is unilateral weakness or paralysis of one vocal fold, phonation will be breathy because the weak fold will not be able to fully adduct to the midline of the glottis. With some patients, a more complete vocal fold adduction may be achieved either when the head is turned toward the affected side or when the larynx is pushed by hand from the affected side (that is, pushed toward the unaffected side). In both instances, the weakened vocal fold can be brought closer to

the opposite fold, thereby improving the quality of the phonation.

Treatments for Prosodic Deficits

Damage to the exterior superior laryngeal branch of the vagus nerve can impair the function of the cricothyroid muscle, which helps vary vocal pitch by stretching and relaxing the vocal folds. Many clinicians and researchers recognize the importance of treating prosodic errors (Darley et al., 1975; Duffy, 1995; Dworkin, 1991; Swigert, 1997). Problems with intonation, stress, and rhythm contribute significantly to the unnatural prosody found in most individuals with all types of dysarthria. The following prosody tasks would be appropriate for individuals with flaccid dysarthria.

- **Pitch range exercises**—Exercises of this type can be a useful starting place for work on intonation. Dworkin (1991) recommended that these exercises begin with an assessment of a patient's ability to perceive obvious pitch changes in the clinician's voice. If the patient is unable to make these distinctions, the prognosis is poor for improving the patient's pitch control. However, if the patient can tell the difference between the pitch changes, the exercises may help. First, have the patient prolong an /a/ at the lowest pitch and then at the highest pitch possible. Once the highs and lows have been established, the patient is asked to sing up and down this pitch range by dividing the range into about eight individual notes. The final exercises have the patient read printed sentences that have arrows written above and below key words indicating the normal pitch changes for those words. For example, an up arrow at the end of a question would indicate that the patient should raise pitch on the final word.
- **Intonation profiles**—This task uses lines to show intonation changes in written sentences. Lines immediately below words indicate a flat intonation. Lines farther below words indicate a drop in pitch. Lines above words indicate a rise in pitch. These lines can be added easily to any written sentence, whether it is a statement or question. Of course, for most patients, it is usually best to start with short and simple sentences and progress to longer sentences. The ultimate goal is to have the patient

take the pitch changes produced in this structured activity and begin to use them in conversational speech.

- **Contrastive stress drills**—These tasks are designed for the clinician to ask a question, with the patient answering it by adding stress on key words to convey the intended meaning of the answer. For example, the clinician may ask the following question about a picture of a man playing football, "Is the man playing basketball?" The patient will answer, "No. The man is playing *football*." The clinician's next question might be, "Is the woman playing football?" The patient's answer to this question would be, "No, the *man* is playing football." A third question might be, "Is the man watching football?" The patient would answer, "No, the man is *playing* football." The length of the questions and the complexity of the pictures for this task can easily be varied to match the abilities of the patient.
- **Chunking utterances into syntactic units**—Duffy (1995) mentioned that some individuals with dysarthria need to learn to divide their utterances according to normal pauses within and between sentences. This is necessary because their dysarthria has limited the number of words they can produce on a single exhalation of air. To compensate for this limitation, the following task teaches the patient to inhale at the points in an utterance where there are natural syntactic pauses. Examples of these natural pauses include after introductory clauses or phrases ["In the morning, (inhale) I went shopping at the store."], between clauses or phrases ["She went there, (inhale) but I missed her."], and between short sentences ["I saw the movie. (inhale) It was pretty good."] By inserting inhalations at points where there are normal pauses in an utterance, individuals with flaccid dysarthria are often able to maintain a more natural rhythm in their speech. This rhythm is lost when the patient haphazardly places inhalations within an utterance.

Damage to the Hypoglossal Cranial Nerve (XII)

Damage to the hypoglossal nerve can result in weakness and reduced range of motion of the tongue, which results primarily in imprecise consonant productions. Treatments for this type of damage to the function of the tongue generally fall into two categories: strengthening exercises and traditional articulation drills.

Strengthening Exercises

As mentioned previously, the value of nonspeech strengthening exercises to treat articulation errors in dysarthria is unclear. Although many such activities are described in the treatment literature, there is little or no evidence of their effectiveness to improve the articulation of individuals with flaccid dysarthria. With this caution in mind, the following four tongue strengthening exercises are provided as typical examples of this type of task. They may or may not be effective in helping patients with dysarthria increase the accuracy of their articulation for speech.

- **Tongue strengthening**—Swigert (1997) described four exercises for increasing the strength of the tongue when weakness appears to be affecting the articulation of lingual phonemes. The first exercise works on tongue protrusion by having the patient push the tongue straight out while the clinician pushes against the tongue tip with a tongue blade. The second exercise concentrates on side-to-side tongue movements by having the patient lateralize the tongue to one corner of the mouth while the clinician pushes it back toward the midline. The third exercise works on tongue elevation by having the patient push the tongue tip upward against a tongue blade held by the clinician. The final exercise concentrates on back of tongue elevation by having the patient push the back of the tongue up against a tongue blade that is inserted into the mouth. Swigert recommended that these four exercises be done while the patient looks in a mirror, so as to enhance the patient's awareness of his or her tongue movements and to increase the patient's monitoring of performance accuracy.

Traditional Articulation Treatment

Traditional articulation treatment tasks concentrate directly on improving the articulation of phonemes. They include a number of principles that have been established components of traditional articulation treatment for many years. Repetitive practice, clinician feedback, and increasing the patient's awareness of articulation errors are all parts of these treatments. Because there are many creative methods of modifying and combining these treatment tasks, beginning clinicians should think of the following descriptions as only templates of how these activities might be implemented. For example, with some patients, it might be very appropriate to combine intelligibility drills and phonetic placement tasks into one treatment activity. Clinicians are encouraged to find which of these activities are best for their various patients.

- **Intelligibility drills**—First mentioned by Yorkston, Beukelman, and Bell (1988), intelligibility drills are tasks in which the patient is given a list of words or sentences to read. Then the clinician turns away from the patient so that he or she will only be able to understand the patient's speech if it is articulated clearly. By not looking at the target word list or at the patient's mouth, the clinician will depend entirely on the patient's articulation to understand the target word. If the clinician does not understand the target word, the patient needs to determine why the word was unclear and then try saying it again. If this second attempt fails, the clinician can look at the target word and give the patient specific feedback on why he or she could not understand the utterance (e.g., "I didn't know it was *sleep* because I couldn't hear the 'l.' Try it again, and let me really hear the 'l' this time.").
- **Phonetic placement**—This procedure treats articulation errors by instructing patients on the correct position of the articulators before they attempt to produce a target sound. Phonetic placement can be especially valuable in that it educates patients on how certain speech sounds are produced. Many individuals with dysarthria realize they are producing speech sounds incorrectly, but they have little understanding of why their productions are in error. For example, phonetic placement can educate dysarthric speakers on why their production of a /d/ actually sounds closer to a /z/ or a /p/ sounds closer to /b/ and so forth.
- **Exaggerating consonants**—Also known as *overarticulation*, exaggerating consonants is a treatment procedure that teaches the patient to *fully* articulate all consonant phonemes. Darley et al. (1975) suggested that most patients need to concentrate especially on medial and final consonants, because these are the sounds most likely to be poorly articulated in connected speech. The improvements in intelligibility can be dramatic when individuals with flaccid dysarthria fully articulate the medial and final consonants in words.

- **Minimal contrast drills**—These drills have the patient concentrate on producing pairs of words that vary by only one phoneme. The distinction between the words can be in the voicing (*park—bark*), manner of production (*dime—mime*), or place of production (*sea—she*). The distinction also can be between vowels (*man—men*), but usually working on consonants does more to enhance intelligibility in most patients. These word pairs can be used alone, in phrases, or in sentences, depending on the needs of a specific patient.

Treatments for Respiratory Weakness in Flaccid Dysarthria

As mentioned earlier, when patients with flaccid dysarthria demonstrate insufficient breath support for speech, it is often difficult to determine if the problem is the result of shallow respiration or the leakage of air at the larynx. When shallow respiration is suspected, there are several procedures that may maximize respiratory function in these individuals.

- **Correct posture**—Many patients have problems with postural support and can be frequently found sitting in their wheelchairs in a slumped position. Their poor postural strength may result in shallow breathing, which often affects phonation and prosody. The simplest strategy to address this problem is to ask the patient to sit more upright. Although this may be successful, reminders to the patient about correct posture will probably be necessary. However, if the patient is unable to improve posture through cues from the clinician, prosthetic devices may be needed to maintain a more upright position.
- **Compensatory devices**—An abdominal girdle that wraps around the waist can help provide the support needed for a patient to maintain a more upright posture. However, this type of device is only a temporary solution for posture problems. Rosenbek and LaPointe (1985) cautioned that prolonged use of such a device may eventually result in pneumonia because it restricts the patient's ability to fully inhale

  Duffy (1995) and Swigert (1997) both described another type of compensatory device that can be used with individuals in wheelchairs. When a padded lap tray on the wheelchair is positioned next to the patient's abdomen, it can provide a rigid surface for the patient to lean on. By leaning forward against this lap tray while speaking, the patient will compress the abdomen and force the diaphragm upward, which may result in a more forceful exhalation for speech.

- **Speaking immediately on exhalation**—Some patients with flaccid dysarthria waste a significant amount of subglottic air by beginning their phonations shortly after they have started to exhale. By cueing the patients to begin phonating immediately on exhalation, they can use more of their available subglottic air pressure. Swigert (1997) suggested that the first step in this exercise is to have the patients place their hand on their abdomen and begin a simple /m/ phonation the moment their hand starts to move inward on exhalation. If necessary, the clinician can place his or her hand on the patient's hand to know when to cue the patient to begin the phonation.

- **Cueing for complete inhalation**—Sometimes breath support for speech can be increased just by reminding the patient to inhale fully before speaking. The clinician will probably need to give frequent reminders about this early in treatment. The ultimate goal is to have these deeper inhalations become a habitual part of the patient's conversational speech. To maximize the efficient use of subglottic air, it is often effective to combine the cues to inhale completely with reminders to speak immediately on exhalation.

SUMMARY OF FLACCID DYSARTHRIA

- Flaccid dysarthria can be caused by any process that damages the lower motor neurons used in speech production. The lower motor neurons are found in certain cranial and spinal nerves.
- The cranial nerves of speech production are the trigeminal nerve (V), facial nerve (VII), glossopharyngeal nerve (IX), vagus nerve (X), accessory nerve (XI), and hypoglossal nerve (XII). The spinal nerves are important for speech production because they innervate the muscles of respiration.
- The speech characteristics of flaccid dysarthria include hypernasality, imprecise consonants, and a breathy voice quality.
- Treatment for flaccid dysarthria can include tasks that attempt to strengthen weakened muscles; however, it may be more productive to work on strategies that concentrate directly on increasing the intelligibility of a patient's speech.

STUDY QUESTIONS

1. Define flaccid dysarthria in your own words.
2. Flaccid dysarthria can occur after damage to which part of the nervous system?
3. Why are lower motor neurons also known as the final common pathway?
4. What are the six cranial nerves of speech production?
5. Which cranial nerve innervates the intrinsic muscles of the larynx?
6. What role do the spinal nerves play in speech production?
7. How can a brainstem stroke cause flaccid dysarthria?
8. How can it be determined if the poor breath support demonstrated by a patient with flaccid dysarthria is the result of weak respiration or poor laryngeal valving?
9. Are muscle strengthening exercises often recommended as a treatment for flaccid dysarthria?
10. What are the two surgical treatments for velopharyngeal incompetence?

C H A P T E R

5

Spastic Dysarthria

(continued)

DEFINITIONS OF SPASTIC DYSARTHRIA

Most definitions of spastic dysarthria mention that it is caused by bilateral damage to upper motor neurons. This is one of the distinguishing features between spastic and flaccid dysarthria, because the latter is caused by damage to lower motor neurons. Most definitions also mention that the speech of an individual with spastic dysarthria is slow, effortful, and has a harsh vocal quality. Of the following two definitions, the one by Parker is unique in that it aptly describes the physical effort many individuals with spastic dysarthria need to apply to their speech.

> [A type of] dysarthria associated with bilateral upper motor lesion and characterized by imprecise articulation, monotonous pitch and loudness, and poor prosody; muscles [can be] stiff and move sluggishly through a limited range; speech is labored and words may be prolonged. (Nicolosi, Harryman, & Kresheck, 1983, p. 80)

> [In spastic dysarthria, the] speech is slow, rasping, labored, and each word is prolonged. It is dominant in lower tones and [sometimes] hardly intelligible. It is like the stiff gait of a spastic paraparetic patient moving with might and main but progressing ineffectually under heavy internal difficulties. (Parker, 1956, p. 163)

NEUROLOGICAL BASIS OF SPASTIC DYSARTHRIA

Spastic dysarthria is a relatively common type of dysarthria, accounting for 9.4% of motor speech disorder cases seen at the Mayo Clinic during a 3-year period (Duffy, 1995). The name *spastic dysarthria* may be a bit confusing to readers who are not familiar with the disorder. It is true that individuals with this disorder have the increased muscle tone of spasticity in various muscles of the vocal tract, but they also have weakness, reduced range of motion, and decreased fine motor control in many of these same muscles. As mentioned, the motor deficits in spastic dysarthria are caused by bilateral damage to the upper motor neuron tracts (Figure 5–1). A clear understanding of the upper motor neuron tracts is important for knowing why spastic dysarthria occurs. Therefore, this chapter begins with a review of the organization and function of the upper motor neurons.

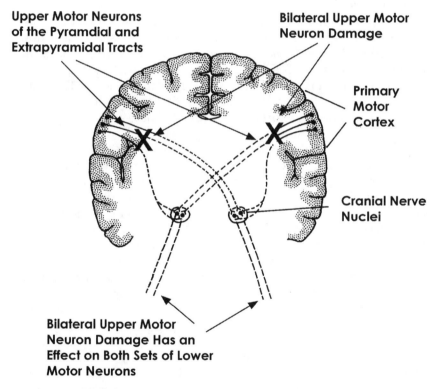

Figure 5–1. Spastic dysarthria is caused by bilateral upper motor neuron damage to the pyramidal and extrapyramidal systems. The "X"s mark lesion site. (Adapted from *Anatomy and Physiology for Speech, Language, and Hearing* [p. 436], by J. Seikel, D. King, and D. Drumright, 1997, San Diego: Singular Publishing Group, Inc. Copyright 1997 by Singular Publishing Group, Inc. Adapted with permission.)

Role of Upper Motor Neurons in Spastic Dysarthria

Whereas flaccid dysarthria is the result of damage to lower motor neurons, spastic dysarthria is caused by damage to upper motor neurons. Specifically, spastic dysarthria is caused by *bilateral damage to both the pyramidal and extrapyramidal neural pathways that serve the speech mechanism.* To better understand how damage to upper motor neurons can cause spastic dysarthria, a brief reexamination of the pyramidal and extrapyramidal systems may be helpful. First, the reader should remember that upper motor neurons are part of the CNS, and they originate in the cortex and brainstem. Second, the reader should remember that upper motor neurons are grouped into the pyramidal and extrapyramidal systems.

The upper motor neurons that are part of the pyramidal system originate principally in the primary motor cortex and course down more or less directly to the lower motor neurons, which, in turn, travel out to the muscles. The upper motor neurons in the pyramidal system are divided into those that travel from the cortex to the cranial nerves (the corticobulbar tract) and those that travel from the cortex to the spinal nerves (the corticospinal tract). The pyramidal system is responsible for transmitting neural impulses for discrete skilled movements down to the lower motor neurons, which then sends them to the muscles. Speech is one of the discrete skilled movements that rely on the proper functioning of the pyramidal system. *Damage to the parts of the pyramidal system serving the speech mechanism will result in weakness and slowness in the speech musculature.* In other words, when the pyramidal system is damaged, the tongue, lips, velum, and other speech structures will demonstrate weak and slow movements.

The other collection of upper motor neurons is called the extrapyramidal system. It is an incredibly complex network of neural pathways. The upper motor neurons in the extrapyramidal system originate primarily in the cortex and brainstem. The extrapyramidal system has numerous interconnections throughout the brain, including the reticular formation and the red nucleus. If the pyramidal system is a direct pathway between the cortex and the lower motor neurons, then the extrapyramidal system is definitely an indirect pathway between the two. Ultimately, however, the upper motor neurons of the extrapyramidal system do synapse with lower motor neurons of the cranial and spinal nerves.

Overall, the extrapyramidal system is responsible for maintaining posture, regulating reflexes, and monitoring muscle tone. The work of the extrapyramidal system is done in parallel with that of the pyramidal system. This means that, while the pyramidal system is transmitting its neural impulses for skilled movement to lower motor neurons, the extrapyramidal system also is transmitting its impulses for posture and muscle tone to the lower motor neurons. When these two systems are intact, their functions blend together remarkably well and allow us to accomplish complex movements effortlessly. When they are damaged, however, a number of problems can arise. As stated previously, damage to the pyramidal system will result in skilled movements that are weak and slow. In turn, *damage to the motor neurons of the extrapyramidal system can result in weakness, increased muscle tone (spasticity), and abnormal muscle reflexes.*

Spastic dysarthria can occur when there is damage to both the pyramidal and extrapyramidal systems that innervate the speech muscles. The co-occurrence of damage to both of these systems is not that unusual, because their neurons are close to each other throughout much of the CNS. In fact, because they are physically so close to each other, damage to one system will almost always cause damage to the other. It is rare to find a stroke, head injury, tumor, infection, or other disorder that causes damage to only the pyramidal system or only the extrapyramidal system. In nearly all instances, the damage will extend to both systems.

Significance of Bilateral Damage

At this point, it should be clear that spastic dysarthria is the result of damage to the upper motor neurons of both the pyramidal and extrapyramidal systems. The final factor leading to spastic dysarthria is that the damage must be bilateral. In other words, the damage must affect both the left and right tracts of the pyramidal and extrapyramidal systems. If the damage is only unilateral, the result will be a relatively mild motor speech disorder known as unilateral upper motor neuron dysarthria (see Chapter 6). Unilateral upper motor neuron dysarthria is not as serious as spastic dysarthria, because most of the cranial nerves serving the speech muscles (except the lower face and tongue) receive bilateral innervation from the upper motor neurons of the pyramidal and extrapyramidal systems. When the damage to the upper motor neurons is unilateral, the cranial nerves will still receive some innervation from the upper motor neurons on the opposite, undamaged side. As a result, most of the speech musculature will be affected relatively mildly, such as is found in cases of unilateral upper motor neuron dysarthria. But when the damage to upper motor neurons is bilateral, many more of the speech muscles are affected, and the result can be spastic dysarthria.

Because both the pyramidal and extrapyramidal systems are affected, the symptoms of this dysarthria are a *combination* of what would be expected if each system were damaged individually. Consequently, the speech production muscles of individuals with spastic dysarthria will show **weakness, slow movements, spasticity** (increased muscle tone), and perhaps **abnormal reflexes**. The weakness and slowness may be most evident in the movements of the tongue and lips, although they certainly can exhibit some spasticity as well. In general, the spasticity probably will be most noticeable in the laryngeal muscles. This spasticity usually will result in hyperadduction of the vocal folds. The spasticity also may affect the velum and cause incomplete velopharyngeal closure during the production of nasal phonemes.

ETIOLOGIES OF SPASTIC DYSARTHRIA

Any injury that causes bilateral damage to the upper motor neurons of the pyramidal and extrapyramidal systems can lead to spastic dysarthria. A number of disorders are capable of creating this type of damage to upper motor neurons. These include strokes, degenerative diseases, infections of brain tissue, and tumors. Because some of the conditions leading to spastic dysarthria are quite rare, the following paragraphs concentrate on the most frequently encountered causes.

Stroke

Strokes are the most common cause of spastic dysarthria. Because of the specific areas that must be damaged (i.e., bilateral damage to both the pyramidal and extrapyramidal tracts), spastic dysarthria will occur only when two or more strokes occur in certain combinations or when a single stroke occurs in the brainstem. The following list highlights circumstances that need to take place before a stroke can cause spastic dysarthria.

- A single stroke can cause spastic dysarthria only when it occurs in the brainstem. This is because the neural fibers of the both the right and left pyramidal and extrapyramidal systems are in very close proximity to each other in the brainstem.

Consequently, a single stroke in the brainstem can be extensive enough to damage both the left and right upper motor neurons of these two systems.

- A single stroke in one of the cerebral hemispheres *cannot* cause spastic dysarthria because it will affect only the left or right pyramidal and extrapyramidal systems, depending on which side the stroke occurs. It takes at least one stroke in each cerebral hemisphere to cause the bilateral upper motor neuron damage that leads to spastic dysarthria.

- A single stroke in one cerebral hemisphere can sometimes *appear* to cause spastic dysarthria. This can happen when a preexisting condition has previously caused damage to the upper motor neurons of the pyramidal and extrapyramidal systems in the opposite cerebral hemisphere. This damage may be an old stroke, head injury, tumor, or similar injury to the other hemisphere. Spastic dysarthria will happen only when the new stroke in one hemisphere is combined with previous cerebral damage in the other hemisphere.

Amyotrophic Lateral Sclerosis (ALS)

Degenerative neurological diseases such as ALS can cause spastic dysarthria. ALS is a disease of unknown etiology that results in the progressive degeneration of lower and upper motor neurons. It is a terminal disorder with an average life expectancy of 22 months from the time of onset. The course of ALS varies across individuals. Some initially have lower motor neurons involvement and demonstrate flaccid dysarthria, weakness in the arms and legs, and muscle atrophy. Other individuals primarily have upper motor neuron involvement in the early stages of the disorder. When the upper motor neuron damage is predominant, individuals with ALS may demonstrate spastic dysarthria, hyperactive gag and jaw reflexes, and swallowing disorders. In nearly all cases, however, the disease eventually involves both upper and lower motor neurons. Once both sets of motor neurons are affected, most individuals with ALS demonstrate a mixed dysarthria of the flaccid-spastic type. Mixed dysarthria is discussed in Chapter 10.

Traumatic Head Injury

A head injury can produce widespread damage to cortical, subcortical, and brainstem structures. In many head injuries, the damage is extensive, because the whole brain is violently shifted within the cranium, which causes linear and rotational movements of the brain in relation to the movements of the skull. The consequences of this shifting can be stretched and torn axons, lacerated brain tissue, and blood vessel hemorrhage in numerous parts of the brain.

Because of this widespread damage to the brain, head injury can cause bilateral damage to the pyramidal and extrapyramidal systems. In such cases, the affected individuals may exhibit spastic dysarthria. It also is likely that a mixed dysarthria, such as flaccid-spastic or spastic-ataxic, will result from a head injury, given the extensive damage that occurs in this type of trauma.

Multiple Sclerosis

Multiple sclerosis is a suspected immunologic disorder that results in the inflammation or complete destruction of the myelin sheath covering axons. The amount of myelin that is affected by multiple sclerosis usually varies from millimeters to several centimeters along the length of a given axon. Multiple sclerosis can affect myelin just about anywhere within the CNS, including the cerebral hemispheres, cerebellum, brainstem, and spinal cord. When there is bilateral involvement of the upper motor neurons, spastic dysarthria may be one of the consequences of multiple sclerosis. However, given the many different areas of the CNS that can be affected by this disease, multiple sclerosis may result in other types of dysarthria, such as ataxic dysarthria or mixed dysarthria. The disorders that can result in a mixed dysarthria are discussed again in Chapter 10.

Other Causes of Spastic Dysarthria

A number of additional disorders can cause spastic dysarthria. For instance, a **brainstem tumor** can affect upper motor neurons similarly to a single brainstem stroke. Because the pyramidal and extrapyramidal tracts are in such close proximity in the brainstem, a single brainstem tumor can compress or destroy the upper motor neurons from both hemispheres and perhaps cause spastic dysarthria. Another condition that can lead to spastic dysarthria is **cerebral anoxia.** This is brain damage from a lack of oxygen in the blood, such as what occurs when an individual stops breathing. As with all of the previously mentioned disorders, cerebral anoxia may cause spastic dysarthria because it is capable of producing widespread neural damage that extends to the upper motor neurons on both sides of the brain. Lastly, **viral** or **bacterial infections** in cerebral tissue also are able to damage upper motor neurons bilaterally. Although these types of infections are sometimes restricted to specific portions of the brain, they also are capable of encompassing much larger areas and, thereby, can affect the upper motor neurons in both hemispheres.

SPEECH CHARACTERISTICS OF SPASTIC DYSARTHRIA

As seen in the definition of spastic dysarthria at the beginning of this chapter, individuals with this type of dysarthria demonstrate a number of different speech errors. Overall, the speech errors in this dysarthria are the result of spasticity, slowness, and weakness in the vocal tract muscles. Articulation, phonation, resonance, and prosody are usually affected more than respiration, but each of these components of speech production can demonstrate the effects of the bilateral upper motor neuron damage. The following paragraphs examine how this bilateral upper motor neuron damage affects articulation, phonation, prosody, resonance, and respiration. Much of the information in this section comes from the Darley et al. (1969a, 1969b) examination of the speech errors of 30 subjects with spastic dysarthria. Table 5–1 lists the most noticeable errors in the speech of the subjects in that study.

Articulation

Darley et al. found that articulation errors were very common in their subjects with spastic dysarthria. **Imprecise consonants** were the most common articulation disorder in that study. It occurred in all 30 subjects with spastic dysarthria. The imprecise production of consonants in this dysarthria may be the result of several factors, including abnormally short voice onset time for voiceless consonants, incomplete articulatory contact, and incomplete consonant clusters (Hardcastle, Barry, & Clark, 1985). **Vowel distortions** also may be heard in spastic dysarthria. (*Note:* Although imprecise consonants are heard frequently in spastic dysarthria, their occurrence is not especially helpful in establishing a diagnosis of spastic dysarthria because these errors are a common problem in every type of dysarthria.)

Table 5–1. The Most Common Speech Production Errors in 30 Individuals with Spastic Dysarthria

Rank	Speech Production Errors
1	Imprecise consonants
2	Monopitch
3	Reduced stress
4	Harsh voice quality
5	Monoloudness
6	Low pitch
7	Slow rate
8	Hypernasality
9	Strained-strangled quality
10	Short phrases
11	Distorted vowels
12	Pitch breaks
13	Breathy voice (continuous)
14	Excess and equal stress

Source: From "Clusters of Diagnostic Patterns of Dysarthria," by F. L. Darley, A. E. Aronson, and J. R. Brown, 1969, *Journal of Speech and Hearing Research*, 12, p. 253. Copyright 1969 by American Speech-Language-Hearing Association. Reprinted with permission.

Phonation

Darley et al. found that **harsh vocal quality** was the most common phonatory error in their subjects with spastic dysarthria. Harsh vocal quality has a definite "friction-of-air" characteristic to it. This harshness occurs when air leaks through a partially open glottis during phonation. In cases of spastic dysarthria, a harsh vocal quality is thought to be caused by the purposeful partial abduction of the vocal folds (Duffy, 1995). By keeping the vocal folds partly abducted, it is thought that individuals with spastic dysarthria are able to prevent the spastic muscle tone in their larynx from closing the glottis too tightly during speech. When speaking, they consequently let some subglottic air leak through their tense, partly abducted vocal folds. The result is a harsh vocal quality.

A **strained-strangled vocal quality** also can occur in spastic dysarthria. A strained-strangled vocal quality is perceptually different from harshness. Compared to the breathy friction of air in harshness, a strained-strangled vocal quality is characterized by subglottic air that is being forced through a narrow, *tightly constricted* larynx. As with harsh vocal quality, a strained-strangled vocal quality is caused by spasticity of the laryngeal muscles, which can result in a tight hyperadduction of the vocal folds. Darley et al. (1969a, 1969b) found a strained-strangled vocal quality to be one of the most distinguishing speech errors of spastic dysarthria. It was more noticeable in this dysarthria than in any other. However, its value as a diagnostic marker is tempered slightly by the fact that it does not occur consistently in all cases of spastic dysarthria. It was present in only 20 of the 30 subjects in that study.

Low pitch is another phonatory characteristic that can appear frequently in spastic dysarthria. It is assumed that the low pitch in spastic dysarthria is a result of increased muscle tone in the larynx. As with a strained-strangled vocal quality, low pitch can be more apparent in spastic dysarthria than in any other dysarthria. However, from a clinical perspective, low pitch alone is probably not distinctive enough to be a consistent indicator of spastic dysarthria because it also can appear in several other dysarthrias.

Resonance

Hypernasality can occur often in spastic dysarthria. Darley et al. (1969a, 1969b) noted it in most of their subjects. It is caused by spasticity in the velar muscles, which slows and reduces the range of soft palate movement. The result is incomplete velopharyngeal closure during nonnasal speech sounds. The hypernasality associated with spastic dysarthria is generally not as severe as that in flaccid dysarthria. The difference between the two is a matter of degree. The hypernasality in spastic dysarthria, while noticeable to a listener, usually does not include nasal emission. In contrast, nasal emission frequently accompanies the hypernasality of flaccid dysarthria, especially in moderate to severe cases.

Prosody

There are several common prosody errors in spastic dysarthria. The first is **monopitch** intonation in connected or conversational speech. It is one of the most obvious characteristics of this dysarthria. It is caused by an overall tenseness of the laryngeal muscles. When these muscles demonstrate this spastic tenseness, they have a reduced ability to contract and relax, which is just the opposite of what is needed normally to vary vocal pitch. For example, the contraction and relaxation of the cricothyroid muscle in the larynx can raise or lower pitch during speech by stretching or tensing the vocal folds. However, when this muscle's ability to contract and relax is restricted by spastic hypertonicity, variations in pitch will also be restricted. The result is a monopitch voice quality.

A second prosody error is **monoloudness**, which is a deficit in the ability to vary vocal intensity during speech. As with monopitch, monoloudness also is caused by increased muscle tone in the laryngeal muscles. Normal loudness variations are achieved by varying the tension of the vocal folds. By increasing and decreasing vocal fold tension, the larynx can precisely regulate the amount of subglottic air that passes through the glottis. Whenever the ability to vary vocal fold tension is reduced, such as in spastic dysarthria, the ability to vary speech loudness will be reduced as well.

Another characteristic of spastic dysarthria is speaking in **short phrases**. Of course, this is a deficit that is most evident in conversational speech. Darley et al. (1975) suggested that short phrasing is probably a natural consequence of speaking through an abnormally tight larynx. The energy expended on forcing subglottic air through hyperadducted vocal folds makes it difficult for individuals with spastic dysarthria to produce utterances of a longer, more normal length. Short phrasing is considered to be a problem of prosody, because the frequent inhalations of air interrupt the normal rhythm of an individual's speech.

Slow rate of speech is yet another prosodic characteristic of spastic dysarthria. It is probably caused by reduced speed and range of movement in the articulators. Weakness in the articulators also may contribute to a slower than normal speaking rate. In addition, Darley et al. (1975) suggested that slow rate may be the result of speaking against tight adduction of the vocal folds, secondary to spasticity in the laryngeal muscles.

Respiration

Problems of respiration do not appear to play as much of a role in spastic dysarthria as they do, for example, in flaccid dysarthria. Much is unknown about how upper motor neuron damage affects the respiratory system. Darley et al. (1975) suggested that there may be some abnormal respiratory movements in individuals with spastic dysarthria. These deviant movements can cause reduced inhalation and exhalation, uncoordinated breathing patterns, and reduced vital capacity. However, Darley et al. also indicated that the phonation and prosody problems in spastic dysarthria are probably more the result of hyperadduction of the vocal folds than any respiratory problems. It would appear then that, if abnormal respiration is present in spastic dysarthria, it is probably "masked" by the more obvious problems of airflow management at the larynx.

Additional Characteristics of Spastic Dysarthria

Several nonspeech characteristics of spastic dysarthria can help in the diagnosis of this disorder. The first of these is pseudobulbar affect. This is uncontrollable crying or laughing that can accompany damage to the upper motor neurons of the brainstem. It appears to be caused by damage to the areas of the brain that are important in inhibiting emotions. In cases of spastic dysarthria or mixed dysarthria with a spastic component, crying is more common than laughing. The display of pseudobulbar affect may be quite independent of the emotions actually felt by the patient. For example, crying may occur during a normally unemotional situation, such as when the name of a spouse or other family member is mentioned in casual conversation. These unexpected displays of emotion can be embarrassing for the patient and distressing for the family. Treatment is limited. Sedatives and antipsychotic drugs have been shown to be ineffective in reducing the emotional outbursts. In some instances, however, pseudobulbar affect lessens in severity as a patient's recovery progresses. Not all patients with spastic dysarthria demonstrate pseudobulbar affect, but it is observed more often in this dysarthria than in the other types.

Although **drooling** can occur in several other dysarthrias, it appears most prominently in spastic dysarthria (Duffy, 1995). It is probably due to impaired oral control of saliva or perhaps to less frequent swallowing. It is not uncommon for affected individuals to claim that their neurological injury has resulted in the production of too much saliva. Although this is unlikely, there are several treatments for this embarrassing and perhaps unhygienic problem. A behavioral approach to treatment works on cueing the individual to consciously swallow more frequently than normal. Pharmaceutical treatments that reduce saliva production also are available.

SPASTIC DYSARTHRIA VERSUS FLACCID DYSARTHRIA

To the untrained ear (and occasionally to the trained ear), the speech characteristics of spastic dysarthria can often sound similar to those of flaccid dysarthria. This may be because these two disorders share many of the same speech characteristics. For example, there can be hypernasality, imprecise consonants, and slow movements of the speech structures in both spastic and flaccid dysarthria. The perceptual similarities between these two dysarthrias is reflected in some of the terms used to describe their symptoms. For example, *bulbar palsy* is a general term meaning atrophy and weakness in the muscles innervated through the medulla (the bulb). This includes the muscles of the tongue, velum, larynx, and pharynx. In fact, *bulbar dysarthria* was once a common name for flaccid dysarthria. The term *pseudobulbar palsy* (a "false" bulbar palsy) means weakness and slowness in the same muscles. This term was sometimes used to describe spastic dysarthria. The distinction between bulbar and pseudobulbar palsy is in their different etiologies. Bulbar palsy is caused by damage to lower motor neurons; pseudobulbar palsy is caused by upper motor neuron damage.

In several ways, however, the symptoms of spastic and flaccid dysarthria can be clearly distinguished from one another. The following is a summary of the more obvious features of the two. This list may help in making a differential diagnosis between these two types of dysarthria.

- Spastic dysarthria is caused by bilateral damage to the upper motor neurons of the pyramidal and extrapyramidal systems. Flaccid dysarthria is caused by damage to lower motor neurons. Be sure to check the medical reports for any information on the site and type of lesion.
- The hypernasality that may be present in spastic dysarthria is usually not as severe as that heard in flaccid dysarthria. In addition, nasal emission is not common in spastic dysarthria but may be quite evident in flaccid dysarthria. Some writers also have described the hypernasality of spastic dysarthria as being more variable and intermittent than that heard in flaccid dysarthria.
- In spastic dysarthria, phonation *can* have a tight, strained-strangled vocal quality, with phonation in flaccid dysarthria having a breathy quality. This can be a very helpful distinction between the two. Remember, however, in spastic dysarthria, a

harsh vocal quality may be heard more frequently than a strained-strangled vocal quality. Do not depend on hearing the strained-strangled quality in all individuals with spastic dysarthria.

- Pseudobulbar affect and drooling are associated more with spastic dysarthria than with any other dysarthria.

KEY EVALUATION TASKS FOR SPASTIC DYSARTHRIA

Duffy (1995) identified three evaluation tasks that are particularly helpful in evoking the speech characteristics most associated with spastic dysarthria. In a comprehensive motor speech evaluation, these tasks should be completed especially carefully if spastic dysarthria is suspected.

1. Conversational speech and reading are useful for assessing the resonance (hypernasality), articulation (imprecise consonants), and prosody (monopitch, monoloudness, reduced stress, short phrases) impairments heard in spastic dysarthria.
2. The alternate motion rate (AMR) task will best demonstrate the slow rate of phoneme production associated with this dysarthria.
3. Vowel prolongation will evoke the phonatory deficits (harsh voice quality, strained-strangled voice quality, low pitch) that are so common in spastic dysarthria.

TREATMENT OF SPASTIC DYSARTHRIA

Depending on the requirements of specific patients, the primary treatment goals for spastic dysarthria might need to target four of the five components of speech production. For example, with some patients it may be necessary to concentrate on decreasing the hyperadduction of the vocal folds (phonation), increasing articulatory precision (articulation), developing more natural intonation in speech (prosody), and decreasing hypernasality (resonance). Respiration is usually not affected significantly in this dysarthria, so the breathing exercises and compensatory strategies mentioned in the last chapter will probably not be necessary. In fact, Duffy (1995) and other writers have cautioned against using the pushing and pulling type of phonation and respiratory exercises, because they tend to increase the force of muscular contractions in the vocal folds. When a patient has hyperadduction of the vocal folds, one of the last things a clinician wants to do is the increase the adduction even further.

Treatment of Phonation Deficits

The harsh or strained-strangled vocal quality in spastic dysarthria is caused by hyperadduction of the vocal folds. Because of the increased muscle tone in the muscles of the larynx, the vocal folds are involuntarily adducted too tightly during phonation. Relaxation and easy onset types of exercises are recommended for this phonatory problem, although there is little if any research demonstrating the effectiveness of such tasks in spastic dysarthria. Indeed, Dworkin (1991) reported that he has had little success in treating vocal fold hyperadduction, but anecdotal reports from other clinicians have sometimes been more positive. As suggested by Dworkin, the following exercises may be most successful with those patients who have mild hyperadduction, but usually all patients with this condition should be given a trial period of treatment nevertheless.

- **Head and neck relaxation**—There are various relaxation procedures for this area of the body. Most of them are based on some type of head rolling motion. One approach is for the clinician to stand behind the seated patient. The clinician tells the patient to relax the neck as much as possible. The clinician then takes the patient's head between his or her hands and slowly, gently tilts it back, then forward, and lastly turns it to the left and right. At the extreme of each position, the clinician holds the head still for about 10 seconds before moving to the next position. A modification of this exercise omits the clinician's hands-on role and has the patient making the motion independently. The clinician talks the patient through the movements. Gentle massage of the sides and back of the patient's neck may also reduce the increased muscle tone in the larynx. Clinicians should consider combining relaxation with the following two phonation exercises. The most logical sequence, of course, would be to begin with the relaxation and then move on to easy onset or yawn-sigh exercises.

- **Easy onset of phonation**—Darley et al. (1975) suggested that vocal quality can be improved by instructing the patient to make softer glottal closures during phonation. The first step is to have the patient exhale while producing a smooth, quiet sigh. Once these soft sighs are produced consistently, the patient is asked to gently initiate a prolonged phonation of an open vowel such as /a/. These prolonged phonations are then shaped into words that begin with vowels or breathy consonant such as /w/. The ultimate goal is to build toward easy phonations of sentences during conversational speech.
- **Yawn-sigh exercises**—This procedure is similar to the easy onset exercise. The patient is asked to inhale slowly while fully opening the mouth, as if yawning. When the inhalation is complete, the patient begins to exhale while producing a gentle, prolonged sigh. The yawning motion facilitates the relaxation of the neck muscles and should reduce some of the hypertension in the larynx. As with easy onset, the sighing phonations are gradually shaped into open vowels, words beginning with vowels or breathy consonants, and finally into sentences and spontaneous speech.

Treatment of Articulation Deficits

The articulation deficits of spastic dysarthria are usually the result of three conditions affecting the articulators: weakness, reduced speed of movement, and reduced range of movement. The primary articulation error in spastic dysarthria is imprecise consonant production. Stretching exercises and traditional articulation tasks are two types of treatments that have been recommended to enhance a patient's ability to more accurately produce consonant phonemes.

Stretching Exercises

It may be beneficial to begin treating the articulation deficits in this dysarthria with gentle, passive stretching exercises. Reducing hypertonicity in the tongue and lips through stretching may result in increased speed and range of tongue and lip movements during speech. Active stretching of the articulators also may increase strength as well. As with the relaxation exercises mentioned previously, little research has examined the effectiveness of stretching as a treatment for spastic dysarthria. Most evidence is anecdotal. For example, in one case study, a patient with spastic dysarthria complained of difficulty with making the articulatory contact needed to produce an /l/ in conversational speech. Shortly after beginning a systematic tongue stretching program, the patient began to demonstrate more rapid and accurate lingual movements for /l/ in all spontaneous speech. Of course, such reports are not from controlled studies, but they should encourage a clinician to try stretching exercises when appropriate.

- **Tongue stretching exercises**—Dworkin (1991) described a series of passive tongue stretching exercises in which the clinician gently grasps the patient's tongue with a gauze pad and carefully pulls it straight forward until resistance is felt. This protruded position is held for 10 seconds. The next steps have the clinician gently pulling the protruded tongue to the left or right sides of the mouth and again holding the position for 10 seconds. Dworkin cautioned against pulling the tongue too forcefully and encouraged the clinician and patient to have patience during these tasks. Active tongue stretching movements by the patient also can be used to increase strength, speed, and accuracy of tongue movements (Duffy, 1995; Swigert, 1997). Examples of these exercises include having the patient protrude the tongue fully, elevating the tongue tip toward the nose, lowering the tongue tip toward the chin, and holding the tongue at the corners of the mouth. Other active tongue stretching exercises include elevating the back of the tongue to the soft palate and pressing the tongue tip into the cheek. *Although these active tongue stretching movements have the benefit of promoting increased strength, they also may increase hypertonicity in some patients.* The clinician should carefully monitor changes in muscle tone. If the active stretching exercises prove to be counterproductive, the passive stretching exercises should be used exclusively.
- **Lip stretching exercises**—In passive lip stretching exercises, the clinician grasps one of the lips gently with a gauze pad and carefully pulls it out and away from the face, holding the position for about 10 seconds. Active lip stretching tasks have the patient making the movements. They include holding a smile, pursing the lips, and puffing out the cheeks. Again, the clinician should monitor any changes in lip muscle tone when active stretching exercises have been recommended. If increased muscle tone is noted, passive exercises should be used exclusively.

Traditional Articulation Treatments

Traditional articulation treatments also are recommended for imprecise consonant productions in patients with spastic dysarthria. These tasks concentrate on increasing the patient's awareness of articulation errors and practicing the best phoneme productions the patient is capable of achieving.

- **Intelligibility drills**—Intelligibility drills are tasks in which the patient is given a list of words or sentences to read. Then the clinician turns away from the patient so that he or she will only be able to understand the patient's speech if it is articulated clearly. By not looking at the target word list or at the patient's mouth, the clinician will depend entirely on the patient's articulation to understand the target word. If the clinician does not understand the target word, the patient needs to determine why the word was unclear and then try saying it again. If this second attempt fails, then the clinician can look at the target word and give the patient specific feedback on why he or she could not understand the utterance (e.g., "I didn't know it was *sleep* because I couldn't hear the 'l.' Try it again, and let me really hear the 'l' this time.").
- **Phonetic placement**—This procedure treats articulation errors by instructing patients on the correct position of the articulators before they attempt to produce a target sound. Phonetic placement can be especially valuable in that it educates patients on how certain speech sounds are produced. Many individuals with dysarthria realize they are producing speech sounds incorrectly, but they have little understanding of why their productions are in error. For example, phonetic placement can educate dysarthric speakers on why their production of a /d/ actually sounds closer to a /z/ or a /p/ sounds more like /b/ and so forth.
- **Exaggerating consonants**—Also known as *overarticulation*, exaggerating consonants is a treatment procedure that teaches the patient to *fully* articulate all consonant phonemes. Darley et al. (1975) suggested that most patients need to concentrate especially on medial and final consonants, because these are the sounds most likely to be poorly articulated in connected speech. The improvements in intelligibility can be dramatic when individuals with flaccid dysarthria fully articulate the medial and final consonants in words.

- **Minimal contrast drills**—These drills have the patient concentrate on producing pairs of words that vary by only one phoneme. The distinction between the words can be in the voicing (*park—bark*), manner of production (*pine—mine*), or place of production (*sea—she*). The distinction also can be between vowels (*man—men*), but usually working on consonants does more to enhance intelligibility in most patients. These word pairs can be used alone, in phrases, or in sentences, depending on the needs of a specific patient.

Treatment of Prosody Deficits

The monopitch, monoloudness, and reduced stress problems in spastic dysarthria may respond to exercises that help the patient regain the vocal tract flexibility that is needed to appropriately vary pitch and loudness. As in nearly all treatment tasks in dysarthria, the general sequence of these tasks is from highly structured activities to more spontaneous procedures that encourage the patient to use the skills learned earlier.

- **Pitch range exercises**—Exercises of this type can be a useful starting place for work on intonation. Dworkin (1991) recommended that these exercises begin with an assessment of the patient's ability to perceive obvious pitch changes in the clinician's voice. If the patient is unable to make these distinctions, the prognosis is poor for improving the patient's pitch control. However, if the patient can tell the difference between the pitch changes, the next set of exercises have the patient prolong an /a/ at the lowest pitch and then at the highest pitch possible. Once the highs and lows have been established, the patient is asked to sing up and down this pitch range by dividing the range into about eight individual notes. The final exercises have the patient read printed sentences that have arrows written above and below key words indicating the normal pitch changes for those words. For example, an up arrow at the end of a question would indicate that the patient should raise pitch on the final word.
- **Intonation profiles**—This task uses lines to show intonation changes in written sentences. Lines immediately below words indicate a flat intonation. Lines farther below words indicate a drop in pitch. Lines above words indicate a rise in pitch. These

lines can be added easily to any written sentence, no matter if it is a statement or question. Of course, for most patients, it is usually best to start with short and simple sentences and then progress to longer sentences. The ultimate goal is to have the patient take the pitch changes produced in this structured activity and begin to use them in conversational speech.

- **Contrastive stress drills**—These tasks are usually designed so that the clinician asks a question, and the patient answers it by adding stress on key words to convey the intended meaning of the answer. For example, the clinician may ask the following question about a picture of a man playing football, "Is the man playing basketball?" The patient will answer, "No. The man is playing *football*." The clinician's next question might be, "Is the woman playing football?" The patient's answer to this question would be, "No, the *man* is playing football." A third question might be, "Is the man watching football?" The patient would answer, "No, the man is *playing* football." The length of the questions and the complexity of the pictures for this task can easily be varied according the abilities of the patient.

- **Chunking utterances into syntactic units**—Duffy (1995) mentioned that some individuals with dysarthria need to learn to divide their utterances according to normal pauses within and between sentences. This is necessary because their dysarthria has limited the number of words they can produce on a single exhalation of air. To compensate for this limitation, the following task teaches the patient to inhale at those points in an utterance where there are natural syntactic pauses. Examples of these natural pauses include after introductory clauses or phrases ["In the morning, (inhale) I went shopping at the store."], between clauses or phrases ["She went there, (inhale) but I missed her."], and between short sentences ["I saw the movie. (inhale) It was pretty good."] By inserting their inhalations at points where there are normal pauses in an utterance, individuals with spastic dysarthria are often able to maintain a more natural rhythm in their speech. This rhythm is lost when the patient haphazardly places the inhalations within an utterance.

Treatment of Resonance Deficits

The hypernasality in spastic dysarthria is the result of increased muscle tone in the velum, which results in slowness and reduced range of movement. Although the hypernasality of this dysarthria is often less severe than that of flaccid dysarthria, it can still be quite evident. As in cases of flaccid dysarthria, treatment can be surgical, prosthetic, or exercise-based.

Surgical and Prosthetic Treatments

As mentioned in Chapter 4, the surgical treatments for hypernasality include a pharyngeal flap and Teflon injections into the pharyngeal wall. Although these are possibilities, the palatal lift remains the more common choice for treating severe cases of hypernasality secondary to spastic dysarthria. However, any hyperactive gag reflex or increased muscle tone of the soft palate can make the use of a palatal lift difficult, if not impossible. Consequently, it is often necessary to decrease velar hypertonicity before fitting a patient with spastic dysarthria with a palatal lift.

- **Decreasing velar hypertonicity**—Dworkin (1991) described a detailed sequence of steps to reduce velar hypertonicity and to simulate the placement of a palatal lift in the mouth. Although the many steps of this procedure are beyond the scope of this book, the initial tasks involve slowly desensitizing the tongue and velum to a foreign object in the mouth. A reduction in velar hypertonicity is achieved by massaging the velum with a tongue blade that is covered by a finger cot. The final step of the treatment sequence is to use the tongue blade to press upward on the velum as if a palatal lift were in place. The reader is referred to the Dworkin textbook for the complete description of this procedure.

Exercise-Based Treatments for Hypernasality

The following treatment exercises for hypernasality may be most successful in cases where the severity is mild. They may also be appropriate for fine tuning velopharyngeal closure after surgical treatment or after a palatal lift has been fitted.

- **Visual feedback**—Although nasal air escape in spastic dysarthria is not as common as in flaccid dysarthria, it may be noted in some patients. If it is present, a mirror can provide visual feedback to the patient regarding any nasal escape of air during the production of non-nasal phonemes. The mirror is held under the nostrils while the patient looks at himself or herself in another larger mirror. The larger mirror provides the patient with a direct view of any fogging of the smaller mirror held under the nose. By trying to minimize nasal escape of air while repeating sentences that contain no nasal consonants, the patient may be able to maximize velar closure. Such simple devices as the See-Scape or a soft feather held under the nose also can provide this visual feedback.

- **Increased loudness**—The perception of hypernasality can sometimes be minimized by having the patient speak more loudly. The louder speech tends to mask the hypernasal quality in individuals with spastic dysarthria. Equally important, the louder speech can often increase intelligibility just by making it easier for a listener to hear what is being spoken. Modeling appropriate loudness levels is a key component of this treatment. Visual feedback on loudness is also helpful for most patients. Such devices as a sound pressure level meter or a Vocalite can give patients a visual cue of what the desired loudness should be.

SUMMARY OF SPASTIC DYSARTHRIA

- Spastic dysarthria can be caused by any process that results in bilateral damage to the pyramidal and extrapyramidal systems.
- In general, the bilateral damage to the pyramidal system results in muscle weakness and slowness in the articulators during speech. The bilateral damage to the extrapyramidal system results in increased muscle tone (spasticity) in the articulators, which may be most evident in the hyperadduction of the vocal folds during phonation.
- The speech characteristics of spastic dysarthria include imprecise consonants, monopitch, reduced stress, and harsh vocal quality.
- Treatment of spastic dysarthria can concentrate on reducing the increased muscle tone by relaxation and stretching exercises. Traditional articulation tasks can target the imprecise consonant productions that are so common in this dysarthria.

STUDY QUESTIONS

1. Define spastic dysarthria in your own words.
2. What nervous system tracts must be damaged before spastic dysarthria can occur?

3. What role does damage to the pyramidal and extrapyramidal tracts play in the symptoms of spastic dysarthria?
4. What is the most common etiology of spastic dysarthria?
5. Why is it impossible for a single hemisphere stroke to cause spastic dysarthria?
6. What was the most common articulation deficit in Darley, Aronson, and Brown's subjects with spastic dysarthria?
7. What is pseudobulbar affect?
8. What do the terms *bulbar palsy* and *pseudobulbar palsy* mean?
9. What is a treatment for hyperadduction of the vocal folds?
10. Describe a tongue stretching exercise.

C H A P T E R

6

Unilateral Upper Motor Neuron Dysarthria

A. Definitions of Unilateral Upper Motor Neuron Dysarthria
B. Neurological Basis for Unilateral Upper Motor Neuron Dysarthria
C. Etiologies of Unilateral Upper Motor Neuron Dysarthria
   1. Stroke
   2. Tumors
   3. Traumatic Brain Injury
D. Speech Characteristics of Unilateral Upper Motor Neuron Dysarthria
   1. Articulation
   2. Phonation
   3. Resonance
   4. Prosody and Respiration
E. Key Evaluation Tasks for Unilateral Upper Motor Neuron Dysarthria

(continued)

DEFINITIONS OF UNILATERAL UPPER MOTOR NEURON DYSARTHRIA

There are fewer published definitions of unilateral upper motor neuron dysarthria than of any other type of dysarthria. One reason for this is the relatively recent recognition of this dysarthria as a motor speech disorder. Darley et al. (1969a, 1969b, 1975) did not classify it as one of the separate dysarthrias, and there were few clinical studies of this disorder before the 1980s. Most of the research into unilateral upper motor dysarthria has been done since the mid-1980s. This is curious because the effects of unilateral upper motor neuron damage on speech production have been recognized for many years (see the 1897 description by Marie and Kattwinkel in Chapter 1).

Be that as it may, the few definitions that are available all mention that articulation deficits are the primary characteristic of this dysarthria. Many also mention that these articulation deficits are almost always mild in severity. The following two quotes are typical descriptions of unilateral upper motor neuron dysarthria:

> Unilateral upper motor neuron dysarthria is a distinguishable motor speech disorder that is associated with damage to the upper motor neurons that carry impulses to the cranial and spinal nerves that supply the speech muscles. It is primarily a disorder of articulation. (Duffy, 1995, p. 222)

> There is . . . demonstrable weakness in the lower face, lips, and tongue on the opposite side [from the lesion] as well as weakness in the extremities of the opposite side. Although unilateral upper motor neuron lesions may . . . be associated with a mild transient dysarthria due to weakness of the contralateral orbicularis oris and tongue, the weakness is usually thought to be too mild to impair speech permanently. (Murdoch, Thompson, & Theodoros, 1997, p. 289)

Although the quote by Murdoch et al. is more of a comment than a definition, it is unique in that it so strongly emphasizes the temporary nature of this dysarthria in many patients. Readers should not assume, however, that all individuals with unilateral upper motor neuron dysarthria will spontaneously recover from the speech deficits associated with it. The effects of this dysarthria can be persistent, and some patients who have it will be appropriate candidates for speech therapy.

NEUROLOGICAL BASIS FOR UNILATERAL UPPER MOTOR NEURON DYSARTHRIA

Chapter 3 explained how upper motor neurons transmit motor impulses from the higher centers of the brain to the brainstem and spinal cord and how these neurons eventually synapse with the lower motor neurons in the cranial and spinal nerves. That chapter also discussed how upper motor neurons are divided into the pyramidal and extrapyramidal tracts. Chapter 5 showed that a key to understanding spastic dysarthria is knowing that both the left and right pyramidal and extrapyramidal tracts must be damaged for spastic dysarthria to result. That is, spastic dysarthria is present only when there is bilateral damage to both of these tracts (Figure 6–1). The damage to the pyramidal system will result in weakness and loss of fine motor control in the muscles of speech production, and the damage to the extrapyramidal system will cause increased muscle tone (spasticity) and abnormal reflexes in many of these same muscles. The combination of these symptoms results in the speech characteristics of spastic dysarthria.

What happens, however, when the damage to upper motor neurons occurs on only one side of the brain (Figure 6–2)? In other words, how is speech production affected by *unilateral* damage to upper motor neurons? Because most of the cranial nerves serving the speech muscles (except the lower face and tongue) receive bilateral innervation from the upper motor neurons, the speech deficits seen after unilateral upper motor neuron damage almost always are less severe than those occurring after bilateral damage. Nevertheless, unilateral damage to the upper motor neurons can cause obvious speech production deficits, despite this bilateral innervation of most cranial nerves.

The most apparent consequences of unilateral upper motor neuron damage are to the muscles of the lower face and tongue. Because the cranial nerves serving these structures are innervated primarily by the upper motor neurons on only one side of the brain, unilateral damage can affect the muscles of the lower face and tongue on the side

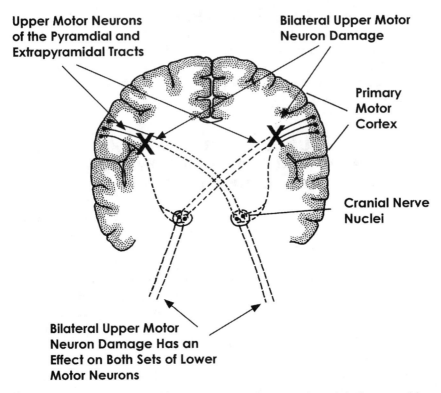

Upper Motor Neurons of the Pyramdial and Extrapyramidal Tracts

Bilateral Upper Motor Neuron Damage

Primary Motor Cortex

Cranial Nerve Nuclei

Bilateral Upper Motor Neuron Damage Has an Effect on Both Sets of Lower Motor Neurons

Figure 6–1. As was discussed in Chapter 5, spastic dysarthria is caused by bilateral upper motor neuron damage to the pyramdial and extrapyramdial systems. The "X"s mark lesion site. (Adapted from *Anatomy and Physiology for Speech, Language, and Hearing* [p. 436], by J. Seikel, D. King, and D. Drumright, 1997, San Diego: Singular Publishing Group, Inc. Copyright 1997 by Singular Publishing Group, Inc. Adapted with permission.)

opposite the damage (Figure 6–3). For example, if upper motor neuron damage occurred on the left side of the brain, the lower right side of the face and tongue might show signs of weakness. In cases of severe unilateral damage, these two structures may be nearly paralyzed on the affected side. More typically, however, this unilateral weakness of the tongue and lower face will usually result in movements that are slow and have reduced range of motion. The tongue might deviate to the affected side when protruded, and lower facial droop may be evident. Patients with these problems often complain that their tongue movements are slow and clumsy.

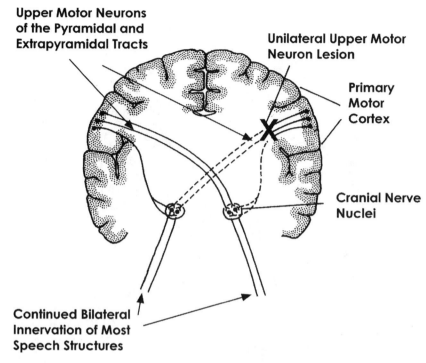

Upper Motor Neurons of the Pyramidal and Extrapyramidal Tracts

Unilateral Upper Motor Neuron Lesion

Primary Motor Cortex

Cranial Nerve Nuclei

Continued Bilateral Innervation of Most Speech Structures

Figure 6–2. Unilateral upper motor neuron damage ("X" marks site) usually will have only a mild effect on speech production because most speech structures will still receive innervation from the unaffected side of the brain. The lower face and the tongue will demonstrate the most significant effects of unilateral damage because these speech structures primarily receive only unilateral upper motor neuron innervation. (Adapted from *Anatomy and Physiology for Speech, Language, and Hearing* [p. 436], by J. Seikel, D. King, and D. Drumright, 1997, San Diego: Singular Publishing Group, Inc. Copyright 1997 by Singular Publishing Group, Inc. Adapted with permission.)

Although the effects of unilateral upper motor neuron damage on the lower face and tongue are recognized widely, the effects of this damage on the other structures of speech production are less clearly defined and less well understood. The traditional view is that because the upper motor neurons bilaterally innervate the velum, pharynx, and larynx, these speech structures should not be affected significantly by unilateral upper motor neuron damage. This is because the upper motor neurons on the unaffected side will provide sufficient innervation to both cranial nerves serving the two sides of these structures.

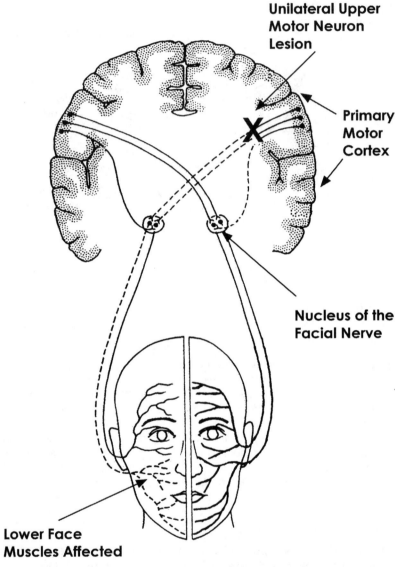

Unilateral Upper Motor Neuron Lesion

Primary Motor Cortex

Nucleus of the Facial Nerve

Lower Face Muscles Affected

Figure 6–3. Unilateral upper motor neuron damage ("X" marks lesion site) will primarily affect only the muscles of the lower face and tongue because most other speech structures are innervated by upper motor neurons from both sides of the brain. (Adapted from *Anatomy and Physiology for Speech, Language, and Hearing* [p. 436], by J. Seikel, D. King, and D. Drumright, 1997, San Diego: Singular Publishing Group, Inc. Copyright 1997 by Singular Publishing Group, Inc. Adapted with permission.)

In reality, however, the clinical picture is not that definite. It appears that unilateral upper motor neuron damage can affect the function of these bilaterally innervated speech structures. For example, some patients with unilateral upper motor neuron dysarthria have a harsh vocal quality. Ideally, this disorder of phonation should not occur in cases of unilateral upper motor neuron damage, because the vagus nerve, which innervates the larynx, receives bilateral innervation. The upper motor neurons on the unaffected side should provide innervation to both sides of the larynx, and vocal fold adduction should be relatively unaffected. However, because the harsh vocal quality strongly suggests some type of laryngeal dysfunction, it would appear that the innervation from the unaffected hemisphere is not a perfect replacement for the innervation from the damaged upper motor neurons in the opposite hemisphere. The question of why some bilaterally innervated speech structures show impaired function following unilateral upper motor neuron damage is discussed again later in this chapter.

ETIOLOGIES OF UNILATERAL UPPER MOTOR NEURON DYSARTHRIA

Any condition that damages the upper motor neurons on one side of the brain can cause unilateral upper motor neuron dysarthria. Moreover, this dysarthria can occur after damage in either the left or right hemisphere. When the damage happens in the left hemisphere, unilateral upper motor neuron dysarthria often co-occurs with aphasia or apraxia of speech. When the damage happens in the right hemisphere, this dysarthria can co-occur with the cognitive and visual deficits associated with injury to that side of the brain. Typically, pathologies that cause focal lesions are the most common cause of unilateral upper motor neuron dysarthria. It is not often associated with degenerative diseases, infections, or metabolic disorders, all of which usually result in widespread neurological damage.

Stroke

Without doubt, the most frequent cause of unilateral upper motor neuron dysarthria is stroke. In a study of 56 subjects with this dysarthria, Duffy and Folger (1986) found that 91% of the cases had been caused by a stroke. Strokes that result in this dysarthria can occur almost any-

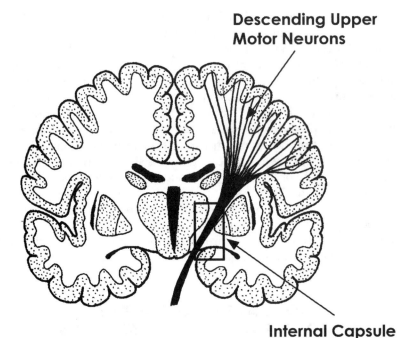

Descending Upper Motor Neurons

Internal Capsule

Figure 6–4. The internal capsule is the point where descending upper motor neurons are squeezed together as they pass between the basal ganglia and the thalamus. Damage to the internal capsule may have a significant effect on motor function, because even a small lesion can damage many upper motor neurons. (Adapted from *Neuroscience of Communication* [p. 176], by D. Webster, 1999, San Diego: Singular Publishing Group, Inc. Copyright 1999 by Singular Publishing Group, Inc. Adapted with permission.)

where in the brain that contains upper motor neurons. This would include many cortical and subcortical areas, as well as the brainstem. Strokes affecting the internal capsule and nearby areas are frequent causes of unilateral upper motor neuron dysarthria. The internal capsule is the point where many descending upper motor neurons are compacted closely as they course downward between the thalamus and the basal ganglia (Figure 6–4). There are several arteries that supply blood to the internal capsule, and even small strokes can have major consequences because of the close proximity of so many upper motor neurons in this area.

Strokes involving the frontal lobe also are leading causes of unilateral upper motor neuron dysarthria. Given the importance of the frontal lobes in formulating and initiating movement, it should not be surprising that unilateral damage to one of them can result in dysarthric speech.

Tumors

Although not a common etiology of unilateral upper motor neuron dysarthria, brain tumors are certainly able to cause this disorder. There are several ways in which a brain tumor can cause the focal, unilateral upper motor neuron damage that results in this dysarthria.

- A brain tumor may directly cause the destruction of nearby upper motor neurons as it grows. This loss of neurons will degrade the transmission of motor impulses from the higher brain centers to the cranial and spinal nerves.
- A growing tumor may displace and "squeeze" upper motor neurons as it becomes larger. This direct pressure from the tumor can compromise the function of the neurons.
- The growing tumor may compress the arteries or veins serving upper motor neurons and interfere with the normal blood flow to or from these cells. The resulting reduction in blood flow would have a negative effect on the function of the neurons.

Tumors such as these could cause unilateral upper motor neuron dysarthria if their effects were restricted to only one side of the brain. However, many brain tumors can have bilateral effects on brain function, even if they are located in only one hemisphere. For example, a tumor in the left hemisphere that caused a generalized increase in intracranial pressure would actually be affecting the functioning of both hemispheres. Such a tumor probably would not cause unilateral upper motor neuron dysarthria because it would have a bilateral influence on brain function.

Traumatic Brain Injury

As with brain tumors, traumatic brain injuries are not a common cause of unilateral upper motor neuron dysarthria. Most traumatic brain injuries result in diffuse damage that affects both hemispheres, because the whole brain is usually stretched and distorted at the moment of impact. As a result, lesions typically occur in both hemispheres following a traumatic brain injury. Nevertheless, it is possible to have head injury where a lesion is primarily restricted to one side of the brain. In such cases, the damage can affect upper motor neurons unilaterally, either at the cortical, subcortical, or brainstem levels. When this happens, it is possible that unilateral upper motor neuron dysarthria may be present.

SPEECH CHARACTERISTICS OF UNILATERAL UPPER MOTOR NEURON DYSARTHRIA

In most cases of unilateral upper motor neuron dysarthria, the effects of the disorder on motor speech production usually are judged to be mild or moderate. This dysarthria is often a short-term disorder for many mildly impaired patients, with recovery occurring over a period of days or weeks. In these milder cases, dysarthria may be the most obvious or perhaps the only indicator that some type of neurological event has taken place (Duffy, 1995). In the more serious cases, unilateral upper motor neuron dysarthria will probably co-occur with other disorders, such as aphasia, apraxia, limb hemiparesis, visual deficits, or cognitive impairments. When there are co-occurring speech and language disorders, it might be difficult to clearly diagnose this dysarthria, because the patient's verbal output could be limited. As a result, the dysarthria may "take a back seat" to these other deficits. Nevertheless, the speech characteristics of unilateral upper motor neuron dysarthria are distinguishable from other dysarthrias and need to be identified accurately during a diagnostic evaluation (Table 6–1).

Articulation

As indicated in the definition at the beginning of this chapter, unilateral upper motor neuron dysarthria is principally a disorder of articulation. This should not be surprising, given that unilateral upper motor neuron damage typically affects the tongue and lower face much more than it does other speech production structures. The most likely cause of the articulation deficits associated with this dysarthria is weakness, reduced range of motion, and decreased fine motor control of the tongue and lips.

Table 6–1. The Percentage of 56 Individuals With Unilateral Upper Motor Neuron Dysarthria Who Demonstrated the Following Speech Production Errors

Percent of Individuals	Speech Production Errors
95	Imprecise consonants
72	Slow AMRs
39	Harsh voice quality
33	Imprecise AMRs
33	Irregular AMRs
18	Slow rate
14	Irregular articulatory breakdowns
11	Mild hypernasality
9	Reduced loudness
5	Strained-harsh voice quality
4	Increased rate of speech in segments
4	Excess and equal stress

Note: from *Motor Speech Disorders: Substrates, Differential Diagnosis, and Management* (p. 228), by J. Duffy, 1995, St. Louis: Mosby. Copyright 1995 by W. B. Saunders Company. Reprinted with permission.

Few studies have examined the speech characteristics of unilateral upper motor neuron dysarthria. One of the most comprehensive was conducted by Duffy and Folger (1986). They found that 98% of their subjects with this dysarthria had articulation deficits. The primary difficulty for nearly all of these subjects was imprecise consonant production. Most of the subjects' articulation deficits had severity ratings in the mild to moderate range. Irregular articulatory breakdowns also were present in some of the subjects but were significantly less common than the problem with consonants. In addition, nearly all subjects had slow AMRs, and 33% had irregular AMRs. The slow AMRs were often so mild that they seldom resulted in slower than normal connected speech rates.

In another study of unilateral upper motor neuron dysarthria, Hartman and Abbs (1992) also found that imprecise consonant productions were a common feature of their subjects' speech. However, the irregular articulatory breakdowns noted by Duffy and Folger (1986) were not evident in this study. The authors attributed this finding to differences between the subjects in the two studies, suggesting that their subjects had more focal lesions than Duffy and Folger's subjects.

Ropper (1987) examined the speech of 10 subjects with unilateral upper motor neuron dysarthria secondary to right hemisphere strokes.

As with the prior two studies, articulatory deficits were the subject's primary speech disorder, with most subjects showing signs of oropharyngeal weakness. As with the results of Hartman and Abbs (1992), the subjects in this study did not demonstrate the irregular articulatory breakdowns that were noted by Duffy and Folger (1986).

Phonation

Several studies have indicated that a mild to moderate **harsh vocal quality** can be present in some cases of unilateral upper motor neuron dysarthria (Duffy & Folger, 1988; Ropper, 1987). For example, Duffy and Folger reported that 39% of their subjects had this harsh quality in their speech. As mentioned earlier, this is a curious phenomenon, because it suggests that the larynx can be affected by unilateral upper motor neuron damage. Conventional thinking has always suggested that most of the cranial nerves are bilaterally innervated by upper motor neurons. Consequently, both the left and right branches of a cranial nerve would still receive full or nearly full upper motor neuron innervation when one upper motor neuron pathway is damaged. In the case of the vagus (X) cranial nerve, which serves the larynx, unilateral upper motor neuron damage should not affect phonation because both sides of the laryngeal muscles are thought to receive adequate upper motor neuron innervation from the undamaged side of the brain.

However, the presence of a harsh vocal quality following unilateral upper motor neuron damage indicates that the function of the larynx is somehow being compromised by the unilateral lesion. Duffy (1995) suggested several reasons for the harshness sometimes noted in unilateral upper motor neuron dysarthria.

- It may be the result of mild vocal fold weakness or spasticity following unilateral upper motor neuron damage.
- There may have been a previous unknown lesion, which combined with a new upper motor neuron lesion on the opposite side of the brain, now causes vocal fold spasticity.
- The harsh vocal quality may be a dysphonia that appears normally in many elderly individuals.
- It may be caused by a general medical condition such as illness or inactivity and, therefore, cannot be attributed directly to the upper motor neuron damage.

Any of these are possible explanations for the harsh vocal quality noted in some patients with this dysarthria. One of the most interesting aspects of this question is the implication that there is still plenty to be learned about how the nervous system controls the speech mechanism.

Resonance

Duffy and Folger (1986) found that 11% of their subjects with unilateral upper motor neuron dysarthria had hypernasality. As with the harsh vocal quality noted in this study, it is surprising to find that velopharyngeal function is affected by unilateral upper motor neuron damage. This is because the vagus nerve, which serves the velar and pharyngeal muscles, is bilaterally innervated by the upper motor neurons. It is likely that the causes of this hypernasality may be related to several of those outlined in the prior section on phonation: general weakness or illness, prior lesions to upper motor neurons in the opposite hemisphere, and so forth. In particular, it may be that the unilateral damage to the upper motor neurons causes a mild muscular weakness in the velum and results in the noted hypernasality.

Prosody and Respiration

Prosody and respiration are rarely impaired in cases of unilateral upper motor neuron dysarthria. Given that this dysarthria is generally a mild to moderate articulation disorder, this should not be surprising. Duffy (1995) reported that when prosody is affected, the most likely cause is a slightly slow rate of speech. The respiration of patients with unilateral upper motor neuron dysarthria is seldom impaired significantly, especially long term. This is probably the result of the widely distributed innervation of the intercostal muscles and the bilateral innervation of the diaphragm. Although some abnormal intercostal muscle movement has been noted in patients with single hemisphere strokes (Przedborski, Brunko, Hubert, Mavroudakis, & de Beyl, 1988), respiration deficits usually are not a problem in cases of unilateral upper motor neuron dysarthria.

KEY EVALUATION TASKS FOR UNILATERAL UPPER MOTOR NEURON DYSARTHRIA

1. As with any dysarthria, the medical records may provide valuable diagnostic information about etiology and site of lesion. Facts about site of lesion can be especially helpful in diagnosing unilateral upper motor neuron dysarthria. As stated earlier in this chapter, it is important to remember that sometimes this dysarthria is the only evidence that a stroke or other neurological event has occurred. The lesion may be too small for neurological imaging procedures to detect, especially early after the onset of the symptoms.

2. Conversational speech or reading a paragraph are useful for evoking the imprecise consonant productions that are so common in this dysarthria. These tasks also can be useful in detecting the irregular articulatory breakdowns that sometimes are present.

3. The alternate motion rate (AMR) task is helpful in highlighting a slowed rate of phoneme production. Remember that in many individuals with unilateral upper motor neuron dysarthria, a slightly slow AMR may not reflect slow connected speech.

4. A prolonged vowel will be useful in detecting the harsh voice quality heard in some patients with this dysarthria.

TREATMENT OF UNILATERAL UPPER MOTOR NEURON DYSARTHRIA

Unilateral upper motor neuron dysarthria presents a few unique situations for the clinician. When it accompanies the language and apraxia deficits of a left hemisphere lesion or the visual and cognitive deficits of a right hemisphere lesion, the relatively mild articulation problems of this dysarthria are often a low treatment priority. The other coexisting deficits almost always are allotted the bulk of treatment time, which is appropriate. The result, however, is that this dysarthria is frequently not treated. On the other hand, when this dysarthria is the only evidence of a neurological pathology (usually a stroke) and there are no obvious language or cognitive deficits, the resulting articulation problems may be so minimal that a clinician may not decide to treat them.

These two circumstances partly may explain the lack of treatment studies on unilateral upper motor neuron dysarthria. Although it is quite understandable that this dysarthria receives little treatment in cases of aphasia and other serious disorders, Duffy (1995) and Swigert (1997) recommended that either strengthening or traditional articulation tasks might be appropriate for many individuals with this dysarthria. They both suggested, however, that the traditional articula-

probably would be more helpful in treating this dysarthria than the strengthening tasks. The following activities are traditional articulation tasks that may be appropriate for individuals with unilateral upper motor neuron dysarthria.

- **Intelligibility drills**—Intelligibility drills are tasks where the patient is given a list of words or sentences to read. Then the clinician turns away from the patient so that he or she will only be able to understand the patient's speech if it is articulated clearly. By not looking at the target word list or at the patient's mouth, the clinician will depend entirely on the patient's articulation to understand the target word. If the clinician does not understand the target word, the patient needs to determine why the word was unclear and then try saying it again. If this second attempt fails, then the clinician can look at the target word and give the patient specific feedback on why he or she could not understand the utterance (e.g., "I didn't know it was *sleep* because I couldn't hear the 'l.' Try it again, and let me really hear the 'l' this time.").
- **Phonetic placement**—This procedure treats articulation errors by instructing patients on the correct position of the articulators before they attempt to produce a target sound. Phonetic placement can be especially valuable in that it educates patients on how certain speech sounds are produced. Many individuals with dysarthria realize they are producing speech sounds incorrectly, but they have little understanding of why their productions are in error. For example, phonetic placement can educate dysarthric speakers on why their production of a /d/ actually sounds closer to a /z/ or a /p/ sounds closer to /b/ and so forth.
- **Exaggerating consonants**—Also known as *overarticulation*, exaggerating consonants is a treatment procedure that teaches the patient to *fully* articulate all consonant phonemes. Darley et al. (1975) suggested that most patients need to concentrate especially on medial and final consonants, because these are the sounds most likely to be poorly articulated in connected speech. The improvements in intelligibility can be dramatic when individuals with unilateral upper motor neuron dysarthria fully articulate the medial and final consonants in words.
- **Minimal contrast drills**—These drills have the patient concentrate on producing pairs of words that vary by only one phoneme. The distinction between the words can be in the

voicing (*park—bark*), manner of production (*dime—mime*), or place of production (*sea—she*). The distinction also can be between vowels (*man—men*), but usually working on consonants does more to enhance intelligibility in most patients. These word pairs can be used alone, in phrases, or in sentences, depending on the needs of a specific patient.

Oral Motor Exercises

Although it may be quite appropriate to treat most individuals with unilateral upper motor neuron dysarthria, there are instances where the articulation errors are so mild that treatment cannot be recommended in good conscience. In this circumstance, the patient may welcome a collection of self-help oral strengthening exercises, such as those in the following section. The clinician can initially instruct the patient on what the exercises are targeting. The patient can then work on them independently. Supportive family members can often be recruited to monitor the patient's performance and progress on the exercises.

Oral Exercise Homework

The instructions to the patient might be something such as the following: "Practice the following exercises 3 times a day for about 10 to 15 minutes. Use a mirror to monitor the correct positions of your tongue, mouth, and lips according to the directions for each exercise."

1. Open your mouth and move your tongue from corner to corner of your mouth. Keeping your mouth open, repeat the full range of motion with your tongue as quickly and as many times as you can. Make sure to touch the corners of your mouth completely each time. Relax and repeat.
2. Slowly open your mouth as much as possible, hold the stretch, then release and slowly close your mouth until your teeth are clenched and lips are tightly closed; hold for 3 seconds. Relax and repeat several times.
3. Open your mouth as much as possible then pucker to form a tight oval with your lips; then relax *just* your lips. Keeping your mouth open, alternately pucker and relax your lips. Repeat several times.

4. Open your mouth and stick your tongue straight out of your mouth as far as you can, then pull it straight back into your mouth as far as you can.
5. Keeping your mouth open, repeat the full range of motion with your tongue as quickly and as many times as you can. Make sure your tongue goes straight out of your mouth and not off to the side. Relax and repeat.
6. Open your mouth and use your tongue to lick all around the lips. Make sure you have continuous contact between tongue and lips and reach all the surfaces of the lips. Relax and repeat.
7. Open your mouth and try to touch your chin with the tip of your tongue; hold for 3 seconds and relax. Then try to touch your nose with the tip of your tongue; hold for 3 seconds and relax. Repeat.
8. Pucker your lips together, making sure the lips are tightly formed together; hold for 3 seconds. Relax and repeat.
9. Smile as widely as you can and hold for 3 seconds. Relax and repeat.
10. Now alternate the pucker and smile; pucker and hold, smile and hold. Make these movements as distinct and completely as you can. Repeat several times.

SUMMARY FOR UNILATERAL UPPER MOTOR NEURON DYSARTHRIA

- As its name implies, unilateral upper motor neuron dysarthria is caused by damage to the upper motor neurons on only one side of the brain. This contrasts with spastic dysarthria, which is caused by damage to the upper motor neurons on both sides of the brain.
- Unilateral upper motor neuron dysarthria is almost exclusively a disorder of articulation. This dysarthria is often present with aphasia and apraxia of speech when the damage occurs in the left hemisphere of the brain. When the right hemisphere is damaged, this dysarthria often co-occurs with the visual and cognitive deficits associated with injury to that side of the brain.
- Treatment of unilateral upper motor neuron dysarthria in-cludes such traditional articulation tasks as intelligibility drills and phonetic placement.

STUDY QUESTIONS

1. Define unilateral upper motor neuron dysarthria in your own words.
2. Why does unilateral damage to the upper motor neurons result in such less severe symptoms in comparison to bilateral damage to these neurons?
3. Unilateral upper motor neuron dysarthria is primarily a disorder of what?
4. What is the most common etiology of unilateral upper motor neuron dysarthria?
5. Why are traumatic head injuries not a common etiology of unilateral upper motor neuron dysarthria?
6. What is the most common articulation disorder in cases of unilateral upper motor neuron dysarthria?
7. What did Duffy suggest as the cause of harsh vocal quality in unilateral upper motor neuron dysarthria?
8. Why are there so few treatment studies for unilateral upper motor neuron dysarthria?
9. Describe intelligibility drills.
10. With what type of patient would self-help oral exercises be appropriate?

C H A P T E R

7

Ataxic Dysarthria

(continued)

DEFINITIONS OF ATAXIC DYSARTHRIA

Damage to the cerebellum is the most common feature in the published definitions of ataxic dysarthria. It is mentioned in nearly all instances. This cerebellar damage results in speech errors that are primarily articulatory and prosodic. These two types of errors often combine to give the speech of individuals with ataxic dysarthria an unsteady, slurred quality. Both of the following definitions are good introductions to ataxic dysarthria.

> [A] dysarthria associated with damage to the cerebellar system and characterized by speech errors relating primarily to timing, giving equal stress to each syllable; articulation problems are typically characterized by intermittent errors ranging from mild to severe; vocal quality [can be] harsh, with monotonous pitch and volume; prosody may range from reduced to unnatural stress. (Nicolosi et al., 1983, p. 79)

> Ataxic dysarthria is a disorder of sensorimotor control for speech production that results from damage to the cerebellum or to its input and output pathways. The dragging and blurred quality of ataxic dysarthria speech has sometimes been likened to "drunken speech." (Cannito & Marquardt, 1997, p. 217)

NEUROLOGICAL BASIS OF ATAXIC DYSARTHRIA

Up to now, this textbook has discussed dysarthrias that are caused by damage to motor neurons. Flaccid dysarthria (Chapter 4) is caused by damage to the lower motor neurons; spastic dysarthria (Chapter 5) is caused by bilateral damage to the upper motor neurons; and unilateral upper motor neuron dysarthria (Chapter 6) is caused by unilateral damage to the upper motor neurons. This chapter examines ataxic dysarthria, which is caused by damage to the cerebellum or to the neural pathways that connect the cerebellum to other parts of the CNS. Incidentally, the term *ataxia* means widespread incoordination and comes from the Greek word for a lack of order.

Although the cerebellum was discussed in Chapter 3, it should be beneficial to review some of the information about it once again. The cerebellum is located below the occipital lobe and is attached to the back of the brainstem (Figure 7–1). It is shaped somewhat like a "small brain," in that it has two hemispheres, a deep fissure between the hemispheres, and a cortical surface of gray matter that has many convolutions. The cerebellum is more complex and fully developed in humans than in any other animal species. This complexity reflects a human's need for very precise muscular control over certain movements, such as for speech.

The cerebellum is a very important part of the motor system. Its primary function is to coordinate the timing and force of muscular contractions so that skilled, voluntary movements are appropriate for an intended task. It accomplishes this by processing sensory information from all over the body and integrating that information into the execution of a movement. The processing and integration function of the cerebellum is obvious, because there are about 40 neural fibers conveying information into the cerebellum for every 1 neural fiber con-

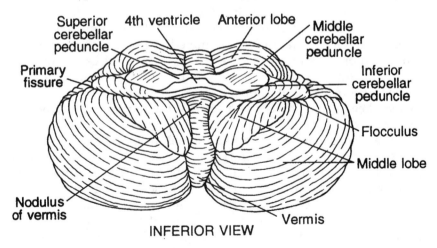

Figure 7–1. An inferior view of the cerebellum. (From *Anatomy and Physiology for Speech, Language, and Hearing* [p. 473], by J. Seikel, D. King, and D. Drumright, 1997, San Diego: Singular Publishing Group, Inc. Copyright 1997 by Singular Publishing Group, Inc. Reprinted with permission.)

veying information out (Brodal, 1992). Although it is not clearly understood how it performs these functions, the general cellular layout of the cerebellum and its neural pathways has been documented in detail.

Neural Pathways To and From the Cerebellum

The cerebellum is attached to the brainstem and communicates with the rest of the CNS through three bundles of neural tracts called the cerebellar peduncles (Figures 7–2 and 7–3). By exchanging information through these neural tracts, the cerebellum is able to monitor ongoing movements and communicate with the cortex concerning planned upcoming movements. Through the first of these tracts (the **inferior peduncle**), the cerebellum receives sensory information from the entire body about the position of body parts, including the eyes, the vestibular system of the inner ear, the joints of the limbs, the skin, tendons, and muscles. This vast amount of sensory information provides the cerebellum with knowledge about the positions of body parts before, during, and after a movement. With this information, the cerebellum is able to recognize what the body is doing during a movement and whether a motor impulse to the muscles is accomplishing the intended result. Overall, this access to sensory information allows the cerebellum to monitor the timing and force of movements while they are being performed. For example, if a body part encounters some unexpected resistance during a movement, the cerebellum detects that resistance immediately through its access to sensory information from the affected body part. The cerebellum can then send adjusting motor impulses to that body part via the superior peduncle (discussed shortly) to compensate for the resistance, thereby keeping the timing and force of the movement appropriate for the task.

The second pathway (the **middle peduncle**) is the largest of the cerebellar peduncles. The neural tracts that travel through the middle peduncle connect the cortex with the cerebellum. These tracts are especially important to the motor system, because it is through them that the cerebellum receives preliminary information from the cortex regarding planned movements. It is thought that these preliminary motor impulses from the cortex are rough approximations of intended movements and need to be coordinated by the cerebellum. The cerebellum coordinates these planned movements by integrating the sensory information it receives from the body with an individual's experience of what the appropriate movement should be. The intended movements are then smoothed and refined according to the current

Basal Ganglia

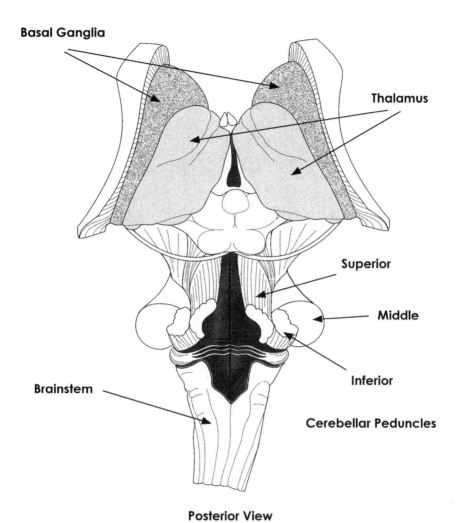

Posterior View

Figure 7–2. A posterior view of the brainstem and cerebellar peduncles. In this illustration, the cerebellum has been removed. (Adapted from *The Speech Sciences* [p. 272], by R. Kent, 1997, San Diego: Singular Publishing Group, Inc. Copyright 1997 by Singular Publishing Group, Inc. Adapted with permission.)

conditions of the body and sent back to the cortex via the thalamus. These processed motor commands are then sent to the motor areas of the cortex, where they are transmitted to the appropriate muscles.

The third pathway (the **superior peduncle**) is the cerebellum's main output channel to the rest of the CNS. There are several destinations for the neurons coursing through the superior peduncle. One of

Pathways Leading to and from the Cerebellum

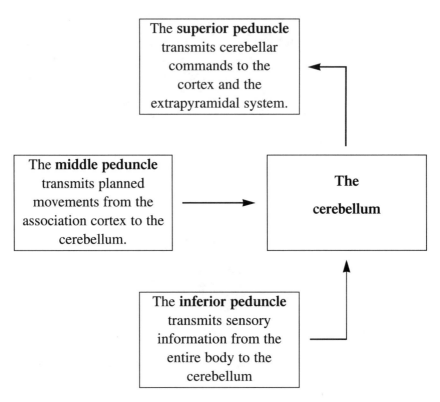

Figure 7–3. A schematic diagram of the neural pathways leading into and out of the cerebellum.

these destinations is the cerebral cortex. It is through the neural fibers in the superior peduncle that the cerebellum sends its processed motor impulses to the motor areas of the cortex, thereby completing the corticocerebellar control circuit. The entire corticocerebellar control circuit therefore starts in the cortex and courses down into the cerebellum through the middle peduncle. The fibers of this neural circuit exit the cerebellum through the superior peduncle and travel back up to the cortex after passing through the thalamus.

Along with the neural tracts coursing out of the superior peduncles to the cortex, there are additional tracts traveling out of the superior peduncle that connect the cerebellum directly to neurons of the extrapyramidal tract. By way of these connections to the extrapyramidal system, the cerebellum can stimulate or inhibit the actions of voluntary muscles. Unlike the neural impulses traveling through the corticocerebellar control circuit, these cerebellar commands to the extrapyramidal system do not travel to the cortex before being sent to the muscles. Instead, these commands take a complex course through the extrapyramidal system as they make their way to the appropriate lower motor neurons. Once these cerebellar motor impulses reach the lower motor neurons, they are then able to coordinate and quickly adjust the movements of the voluntary muscles according to the changing positions and circumstances of the body.

Incidentally, the neurons that course through these three cerebellar pathways are called **cerebellar control circuits**, not upper motor neurons. Although they do transmit motor impulses, these neurons do not actually synapse with lower motor neurons, which, by definition is what upper motor neurons do. Most neurons coursing out of the cerebellar peduncles synapse with either true upper motor neurons (primarily those of the extrapyramidal system) or interneurons in the brainstem and spinal cord.

THE CEREBELLUM AND SPEECH

Without doubt, the cerebellum plays an important role in coordinating the many intricate muscular contractions needed to produce intelligible speech. However, the precise nature of the cerebellum's influence on speech is unclear. There are probably at least two ways in which the cerebellum influences speech movements. One of these is through the corticocerebellar control circuit discussed previously. The planned motor impulses of a planned speech act are sent from the cortex to the cerebellum. The cerebellum coordinates and refines these preliminary speech movements according to (a) sensory information about the positions and conditions of the articulators and (b) prior practice on what the skilled target movement should be. These coordinated motor impulses are then sent to the thalamus for additional refinement and then forwarded on to the motor cortex. From there, the motor impulses are transmitted to the appropriate muscles for speech production.

Another way in which the cerebellum may influence speech movements is through its connections to the extrapyramidal system. As described in the preceding section of this chapter, the cerebellum can make rapid adjustment in the timing and force of movements to compensate for unexpected change in the circumstances of a movement.

For example, if someone is attempting to talk with food in his or her mouth, the cerebellum will detect that tongue movements are being slowed by the presence of the food. To maintain intelligible articulation of speech sounds, the cerebellum will adjust the firing of the appropriate motor neurons to the tongue so that intelligible articulation can be maintained despite this resistance to tongue movement during speech.

Because of this remarkable dual ability to coordinate and modify both planned and ongoing speech movements, the cerebellum is a key player in the motor speech system. However, because it is so important, damage to the cerebellum or to its control circuits may significantly harm an individual's ability to produce normal speech.

ETIOLOGIES OF ATAXIC DYSARTHRIA

Damage to different parts of the cerebellum or its control circuits can result in a variety of movement disorders. In general, individuals with cerebellar damage have problems coordinating their voluntary movements. It seems as if they have trouble controlling the timing and force of their movements, especially at the beginning and ending of an action. For example, their movements may be wavering and jerky when reaching to pick up an object. This jerky unsteadiness indicates that the range and direction of movements also can be affected by cerebellar damage. Altogether, these movement deficits of timing, force, range, and direction are known as **cerebellar ataxia**.

Impairment of equilibrium during walking can be one of the more obvious symptoms of cerebellar damage. In these cases, individuals walk with a wide-based and staggering gait, frequently giving the impression that they are just about to fall. Cerebellar damage also can cause deficits in voluntary eye movements, intention tremors, hypotonia of the muscles, and problems with motor learning.

Because there is so much about the operation of the cerebellum that is unknown, neuroscientists are unclear about how different types of cerebellar damage affect speech production. Darley et al. (1975) stated that ataxic dysarthria often occurs when there is generalized or bilateral damage to the cerebellum. They also reported that speech coordination might be especially dependent on a part of the cerebellum at the midpoint between the cerebellar hemispheres called the **vermis** (see Figure 7–1). Recent research has suggested that focal lesions also can cause ataxic dysarthria. Duffy (1995) cited several studies suggesting that ataxic dysarthria can be caused by focal damage to the superior peduncle, the lateral portions of the cerebellar hemispheres, or areas near the vermis.

Degenerative Diseases

There are a number of degenerative disorders that result in progressive cerebellar dysfunction and are frequent causes of ataxic dysarthria. **Autosomal dominant cerebellar ataxia of late onset** is a hereditary disease that usually begins in middle age. Ataxic dysarthria is only one of many features that may be present in this disorder. Progressive cerebellar ataxia, retinal degeneration, muscle rigidity, sensorineural deafness, balance deficits, dementia, and a number of other neurological features also may be evident. The presence of these symptoms can vary significantly among individuals with this disease, even among affected members of the same family. It is a terminal disease, with death usually occurring within several years of the first appearance of symptoms.

Idiopathic sporadic late-onset cerebellar ataxia is a similar disease, except that it usually does not include as many neurological symptoms. It often results only in progressive cerebellar ataxia, ataxic dysarthria, and balance deficits. This disorder also tends to begin in middle age. As its name suggests, the cause of idiopathic sporadic late-onset cerebellar ataxia is unknown.

Friedreich's ataxia is a progressive hereditary disease that can affect the spinal cord as well as the cerebellum and is accordingly classed as a spinocerebellar disease. Although often described as a common cause of cerebellar ataxia, it is actually a rare disorder with a prevalence of only 2 per 100,000. The symptoms of Friedreich's ataxia, which usually become evident when individuals are in their 20s, include cerebellar ataxia affecting gait and manual dexterity, dysarthria, and visual disorders. The less common symptoms include dementia and sensorineural deafness. Few people with this disorder survive past their 40s, with death often occurring after coma or heart failure. The dysarthria associated with Friedreich's ataxia is not necessarily purely ataxic in nature, because this disorder does not usually affect only the cerebellum and its control circuit. There also can be evidence of lower motor neuron weakness and certain signs of extrapyramidal system involvement. Because these other areas of the motor system can be affected, the dysarthria associated with Friedreich's ataxia is often of a mixed type, which is examined in Chapter 10.

Olivopontocerebellar degeneration is another progressive cerebellar disorder that tends to run in families. This disorder results in atrophy of the middle cerebellar peduncle, much of the cerebellum, and parts of the pons. One of the primary symptoms of olivoponto-cerebellar degeneration is cerebellar ataxia. The neuron degeneration associated with this disorder also can involve the basal ganglia and some of the corticospinal tract. Symptoms of a parkinsonian nature, such as muscular rigidity and reduced range of movement, also are often present. As with Friedreichs ataxia, the dysarthria associated with olivopontocerebellar degeneration may usually be more mixed in nature than a pure ataxic type.

Stroke

As with the other areas of the brain, the cerebellum has a rich arterial blood supply. There are several arteries serving the cerebellum, includ-ing the superior cerebellar artery and the anterior inferior cerebellar artery. Blockage of blood flow through either of these arteries can cause ataxic dysarthria. Ruptured aneurysms or arteriovenous malforma-tions in these arteries also have been linked to ataxic dysarthria. In fact, about 10% of intracerebral hemorrhages primarily affect the cerebel-lum or the neurons in the cerebellar control circuits (Heilman, Watson, & Greer, 1977). Most cerebellar stokes result in the sudden onset of a number of "cerebellar signs," including limb ataxia, problems with bal-ance, visual deficits, and ataxic dysarthria.

Toxic Conditions

Different toxic and metabolic conditions can affect the functioning of the cerebellum. The toxic conditions that have been associated with cerebellar dysfunction include lead and mercury poisoning, chronic and acute consumption of alcohol, and exposure to such chemicals as acrylamide and cyanide. Most of these conditions are treatable, and any instances of ataxic dysarthria, if present, will usually resolve as the toxic levels of these substances decrease. Toxic levels of phenytoin (Dilantin), an antiseizure drug, also have been associated with ataxic dysarthria. Unlike many of the other toxic conditions, the effects of long-term phenytoin overdosage may be irreversible.

Some of the metabolic conditions that can result in cerebellar dys-function include prolonged vitamin E or B_{12} deficiency, severe cases of hypothyroidism, and such hereditary disorders as Wilson's disease. Each of these can cause ataxic dysarthria, although they are not common disorders. Incidentally, Wilson's disease usually results in mixed dysarthria and is discussed in more detail in Chapter 10.

Traumatic Head Injury

Cerebellar tissue can be distorted and stretched by the force of head trauma and can be just as susceptible to the dynamics of an impact as the other parts of the brain are. As with most head injuries, traumatic damage to the cerebellum tends to be diffuse. However, the cerebellar peduncles are especially vulnerable to the twisting and rotational forces of such an injury, because the cerebellum is essentially an appendage that is attached to the brainstem. During a rapid rotational movement of the head, some of the highest amounts of axon stretching may be at these points of attachment. As a result, the axons coursing through the peduncles often are especially susceptible to damage during a head injury.

Tumors

Tumors can affect cerebellar function in several ways. First, a tumor may grow in cerebellar tissue, directly destroying cells and compressing the cerebellum if it grows large enough. Second, a tumor may grow near the cerebellum, for example, on the occipital lobe, which then compresses cerebellar tissue. Third, a brainstem tumor may interfere with the functions of the cerebellar control circuits. The appearance of ataxic dysarthria following a cerebellar tumor depends on the location and size of the tumor. Duffy (1995) reported that tumors accounted for about 3% of the cases of ataxic dysarthria at the Mayo Clinic over a 21-year period.

There are certain types of tumors that tend to appear frequently in the cerebellum. **Metastatic tumors** are among the most common. These tumors are formed when one tumor (the primary tumor) sheds cancerous cells that seed a secondary (metastatic) tumor in another part of the body. Primary metastatic cerebellar tumors are usually located in such sites as the skin (melanomas), lungs, kidneys, or breasts. A slow-growing type of tumor called a **low-grade astrocytoma** can appear frequently in the cerebellum, especially in children. More than 50% of these tumors in children are located in the cerebellum. When it occurs in adults, this type of tumor usually appears between the ages of 30 to 60. **Hemangioblastomas** are benign tumors of proliferated blood vessels found occasionally in the cerebellum. The symptoms of a hemangioblastoma usually appear late in childhood, but sometimes they are not evident until the affected individual is an adult. Progressive cerebellar ataxia and ataxic dysarthria can be among the symptoms of a cerebellar hemangioblastoma.

Other Possible Etiologies

Although they are not the most common causes of cerebellar dysfunction, ataxic dysarthria also can result from:

- Viral infections that invade the cerebellum.
- Other infections, such as trichinosis, typhus, and syphilis that may affect cerebellar functions.
- A bacterial abscess (a localized collection of pus) near the cerebellum that may compress the surrounding brain tissue. Such an abscess will probably present symptoms similar to those of a cerebellar tumor.

SPEECH CHARACTERISTICS
OF ATAXIC DYSARTHRIA

In general, individuals with ataxic dysarthria give the impression that the movements of their speech mechanism are poorly coordinated. As in other cerebellar-based movement problems, patients with ataxic dysarthria seem to have problems controlling the timing and force of the many muscular contractions that are needed to produce clearly articulated speech. It is often reported that individuals with ataxic dysarthria have a drunken quality in their speech. There are frequent complaints that articulation is slurred and prosody is monotonous. Such complaints reflect Duffy's (1995) statement that ataxic dysarthria "is predominantly an articulatory and prosodic disorder" (p. 153). Some medical professionals use the term *scanning speech* to describe ataxic dysarthria. In that usage, this term describes how individuals with this dysarthria often demonstrate a slow, deliberate production of syllables, with each syllable in a word receiving equal stress.

Articulation

Articulation deficits are a significant problem in ataxic dysarthria. Darley et al. (1969a, 1969b) found that **imprecise consonant articulation** was the most prevalent speech error in this type of dysarthria (Table 7–1). Another common characteristic is **distorted vowels**. It is

Table 7–1. The Most Common Speech Production Errors in 30 Individuals With Ataxic Dysarthria

Rank	Speech Production Errors
1	Imprecise consonants
2	Excess and equal stress
3	Irregular articulatory breakdown
4	Distorted vowels
5	Harsh voice quality
6	Prolonged phonemes
7	Prolonged intervals
8	Monopitch
9	Monoloudness
10	Slow rate

Source: From "Clusters of Diagnostic Patterns of Dysarthria," by F. L. Darley, A. E. Aronson, and J. R. Brown, 1969, *Journal of Speech and Hearing Research, 12*, p. 256. Copyright 1969 by American Speech-Language-Hearing Association. Reprinted with permission.

the imperfect articulation of phonemes that gives ataxic dysarthria its characteristic slurred quality. These distortions are caused by cerebellar damage that disrupts the timing, force, range, and direction of movements needed to maintain normal articulation. Such deficits in the performance of complex movements requiring more than one body part are sometimes called **decomposition of movement**.

The articulation errors in ataxic dysarthria, however, may not always be consistent. Some individuals with ataxic dysarthria also may demonstrate **irregular articulatory breakdowns**, meaning that their imprecise consonant and vowel productions can vary from utterance to utterance. These intermittent breakdowns will usually occur most frequently in sentences that contain several multisyllabic words, but the errors may not appear on every production of such a sentence. The breakdowns often give the appearance that the syllables are being compressed during the production of a word. Incidentally, hyperkinetic dysarthria (Chapter 9) is the only other dysarthria in which irregular articulatory breakdowns may be present, although Duffy and Folger (1986) did find it in a few of their subjects with unilateral upper motor neuron dysarthria. In general, the articulation errors in most of the other dysarthrias tend to be quite consistent during speech (Darley et al., 1975).

Prosody

Prosodic errors also are prominent in ataxic dysarthria. At least six prosodic deficits can be present in the speech of individuals with this type of dysarthria:

- Equal and excess stress
- Prolonged phonemes
- Prolonged intervals between phonemes
- Monopitch
- Monoloudness
- Slow rate.

Darley et al. (1969a, 1969b) ranked each of these within the top 10 most deviant speech characteristics of their subjects with cerebellar lesions.

Equal and excess stress is the tendency of many speakers with ataxic dysarthria to put equal stress on syllables or words that would normally have varied stress patterns. At the same time, some speakers with ataxic dysarthria also tend to put excessive stress on syllables or words that are not normally stressed to that degree. This stress pattern can be a distinguishing characteristic of ataxic dysarthria. When listening to an individual speaking in this manner, the syllable stress on such words as *record* (the noun) and *record* (the verb) might appear to be quite similar, with the listener needing to infer the correct word from the context. This stress pattern gives the impression that each syllable or word is produced separately, without one part of a word or sentence being influenced by the others.

The next two prosodic errors, **prolonged phonemes** and **prolonged intervals between phonemes**, are related. One of the hallmarks of cerebellar damage is slow movement on both single and repetitive motion tasks. This slowness includes the movements of the speech musculature, resulting in a slowed production of phonemes and a lengthening of the intervals between phonemes. Netsell and Kent (1975) indicated that these prolongations are probably caused by decreased muscle tone (hypotonia). They suggested that this hypotonia results in a general slowness in the contractions of the speech muscles, resulting in an overall prolongation of speech production. Naturally, these prolongations of phonemes and intervals contribute to a **slow rate** of speech, which is another prosodic defect that is very common in ataxic dysarthria.

Darley et al. (1969a, 1969b) noted **monopitch** and **monoloudness** in 20 and 18 of their 30 subjects with cerebellar damage, respectively. They suggested that these two prosodic errors also are caused by hypotonia of the speech muscles. It is logical to assume that the equalizing of stress also contributes to the perception of these two characteristics in individuals with ataxic dysarthria.

Phonation

Few phonatory deficits are usually noted in ataxia dysarthria. Darley et al. (1969a, 1969b) found that **harsh voice quality** is certainly the most prominent phonatory deficit that may be evident in this dysarthria. They identified this phonatory problem in 21 of their 30 subjects. These researchers suggested that this condition is caused by decreased muscle tone in the laryngeal and respiratory structures, which prevents the full contraction of these muscle groups.

Another phonatory problem in ataxic dysarthria can be **voice tremor**. Cerebellar damage may cause tremors that affect various body parts, and when the laryngeal or respiratory muscles are involved, the result can be a distinguishable voice tremor. Although not common, it can been observed in some individuals with this dysarthria (Ackermann & Ziegler, 1991; Darley et al. (1969a, 1969b).

Resonance

Hypernasality is seldom a serious problem in ataxic dysarthria. Darley et al. (1969a, 1969b) did not rank it as one of the significant speech errors in their study of subjects with cerebellar lesions, although 10 of their 30 subjects demonstrated some instances of it. These researchers, nevertheless, concluded that it is not a prominent characteristic of this dysarthria. Duffy (1995) also reported that abnormal resonance is infrequent, but he noted that intermittent *hypo*nasality may be evident in some individuals, probably because of timing errors between the muscles of the velum and the other muscles of articulation.

Respiration

Cerebellar damage can cause uncoordinated movements in the respiratory muscles, which can contribute to the speech deficits heard in ataxic dysarthria. Although few studies have examined the respiration of individuals with ataxic dysarthria, several have shown that respiration during speech can contain **exaggerated or paradoxical movements** (Luchsinger & Arnold, 1965; Murdoch, Chenery, Stokes, & Hardcastle, 1991). Paradoxical movements occur when different muscle groups work against each other rather than in coordination. Naturally, such abnormal respiratory movements can affect speech production. Exaggerated movements of the respiratory muscles can lead to excessive loudness variations during many speech tasks, including conversation.

Paradoxical movements of the intercostal muscles and the diaphragm can reduce the vital capacity of the lungs and thereby limit the amount of subglottic air available for speech. Insufficient subglottic air pressure during conversational speech often leads the affected individual to speak on residual air. This, in turn, can lead to an increased rate of speech, decreased loudness, and a harsh vocal quality. Ultimately, these abnormal respiratory movements can affect the prosody of individuals with ataxic dysarthria. Incidentally, Darley et al. (1969a, 1969b) did not notice any rapid involuntary inhalations or exhalations of air in their subjects with ataxic dysarthria. Such involuntary respiratory movements are observed much more frequently in cases of hyperkinetic dysarthria (Chapter 9).

KEY EVALUATION TASKS FOR
ATAXIC DYSARTHRIA

1. Speech AMRs can be one of the most valuable evaluation tasks when ataxic dysarthria is suspected. The overall rate will probably be slower than normal. In addition, many individuals with this dysarthria will be unable to maintain a steady rhythm as they repeat the target sounds. In the most severe cases, they may speed up abruptly and then, just as unexpectedly, slow down during this speech production task. Their difficulty in maintaining a regular rhythm highlights how cerebellar damage can affect the timing of movements by different muscle groups.

2. Reading, conversational speech, and repeating sentences containing numerous multisyllabic words also are important evaluation tasks (Duffy, 1995). The complexity of these longer speech activities will reveal any inaccurate speech movements. As such, they can be especially effective at evoking the irregular articulatory breakdowns that often appear in ataxic dysarthria. Remember that these breakdowns tend to occur more frequently on multisyllabic words than on words of shorter length. Furthermore, these three tasks should reveal any prosodic errors that may be present in connected speech.

TREATMENT OF ATAXIC DYSARTHRIA

As stated previously, ataxic dysarthria is the result of damage to the cerebellum or the cerebellum control circuit. This damage often affects the speed, force, and timing of movements by the articulators, which results in movements that are typically described as "uncoordinated." In a majority of instances, the most evident speech errors in this dysarthria are those related to articulation and prosody.

Respiration

Most patients with ataxic dysarthria do not need to work on strengthening their respiration abilities. Rather, they usually should concentrate on controlling their airflow more accurately during speech. The uncoordinated movements of their respiratory muscles can leave them speaking on residual air, which affects prosody and phonation. There are numerous tasks that may be useful in helping these patients gain better breath control during speech.

- **Slow and controlled exhalation**—In this simple task, the patient is asked to inhale fully and then exhale in a slow, steady stream. Using a stopwatch, the clinician times the length of the exhalation. The goal is to increase the length and steadiness of the airflow over several sessions. Dworkin (1991) described an advanced variation on this task in which the patient is asked to inhale fully, begin a slow exhalation for 3 seconds, stop the exhalation by holding the breath for about 1 second, then continuing with the exhalation. The difficulty of this task can be increased until the patient is holding and releasing the air three times on a single breath.
- **Speak immediately on exhalation**—Because of poor coordination of the respiratory and laryngeal muscles, many patients with ataxic dysarthria waste a significant amount of their subglottic air by beginning their phonations a second or two after they have started to exhale. The task of speaking immediately on exhalation concentrates on making sure patients initiate phonation the moment they begin an exhalation. Swigert (1997) suggested that the patient place a hand on the abdomen and begin a simple /m/ phonation the moment the hand starts to move inward on the exhalation. The clinician can place his or her hand on the patient's hand

to know when to cue the patient to begin the phonation, if necessary.

- **Stop phonation early**—Because individuals with ataxic dysarthria often demonstrate shallow respiration, they may try to speak for a longer period than their limited subglottic air supply allows. This results in speaking on residual air and frequently leads to harsh vocal quality, decreased loudness, and increased rate of speech. Consequently, it is often necessary for the patient to learn to end an utterance before running low on air. This can often be initially accomplished by having the clinician provide verbal and visual cues that tell the patient when to stop phonating and take another breath. Over time, as the patient becomes more independent at stopping phonation before speaking on residual air, the clinician's cues can be faded.

- **Optimal breath group**—This task is somewhat similar to the stopping phonation early procedure. The optimal breath group task teaches the patient how many syllables or words can be said clearly on one full inhalation (Linebaugh, 1983). Once a baseline has been established, the patient can work on increasing the length of the breath group, perhaps through deeper inhalations, more controlled exhalations, or beginning phonations immediately on exhalation. The optimal breath group task is similar to the cued reading materials and chunking utterances into syntactic units tasks, which will be described shortly.

Prosody

The prosodic problems experienced by individuals with ataxic dysarthria usually involve rate, stress, and intonation. By slowing their rate, these individuals often can improve their intelligibility. By incorporating more typical stress and intonation into their utterances, their speech may exhibit a more natural quality.

Rate Control

Although a slow or irregular rate of speech is characteristic of ataxic dysarthria, many individuals with this disorder still attempt to speak at a rate that is too rapid for their speech production capabilities. By speaking too rapidly, they do not give their articulators sufficient time to reach target positions, nor do they give a listener enough time to assimilate the spoken message. The amount of slowing needed to improve intelligibility does not always have to be significant. Often minimal decreases in rate can result in noticeably more understandable speech. The following rate control tasks are some of the procedures that may successfully slow the speaking rate of individuals with ataxic dysarthria. These tasks are highly structured and are probably most appropriate for the initial treatment steps in which increasing a patient's awareness of a slower, more intelligible rate is the primary goal.

- **Reciting syllables to a metronome**—Dworkin (1991) suggested using a metronome to set the pace of syllable production. In this task, the metronome is set to the appropriate rate, and the patient is asked to recite or read familiar passages such as the Pledge of Allegiance, a well-known poem, or something similar. The patient should produce one syllable for every beat of the metronome. Although the resulting speech will sound automated, this is acceptable because the goal in this task is to build the patient's awareness of a more appropriate speech rate. Naturally, use of the metronome is discontinued as the slower rate of speech is independently incorporated into the patient's utterances.
- **Finger or hand tapping**—Finger or hand tapping can be substituted for a metronome to set the pace of appropriate syllable production. Initially, the clinician sets the pace by tapping with a finger or hand, with the patient following the tempo while reading a familiar passage. Once the pace is established, the patient can try to do the tapping. Be aware, however, that the typically uncoordinated movements of such a patient may make it very difficult for him or her to maintain a regular pace when trying to tap independently.
- **Cued reading material**—Various rate cueing techniques can be used with written sentences or paragraphs. One type of cueing is to have the clinician point to a word or syllable at the desired rate, and the patient is asked to read the material at that pace. Another type of cueing is to have reading material that has slash marks or spaces to indicate when pauses are necessary while reading aloud. For example, a prepared sentence from a story may look like this: "With a feeling of deep /// yet most singular affection /// I regarded my friend." At the slash marks, the patient should pause for a brief moment

before continuing to read. Such reading materials also can be a useful tool in introducing a patient to the optimal breath group duration tasks that were discussed in the section on respiration deficits. They may also be useful for introducing patients to the task of chunking utterances into syntactic units (discussed shortly).

Stress and Intonation

Stress and intonation exercises for individuals with ataxic dysarthria should concentrate on developing more natural pitch and loudness variations in connected speech. The following tasks might be appropriate for the initial steps of a treatment plan that addresses the stress and intonation problems of patients with ataxic dysarthria.

- **Contrastive stress drills**—These tasks are usually designed so that the clinician asks a question, and the patient answers it by adding stress on key words to convey the intended meaning of the answer. For example, the clinician may ask the following question about a picture of a man playing football, "Is the man playing basketball?" The patient will answer, "No. The man is playing *football.*" The clinician's next question might be, "Is the woman playing football?" The patient's answer to this question would be, "No, the *man* is playing football." The length of the questions and the complexity of the pictures for this task can easily be varied according to the abilities of the patient.
- **Pitch range exercises**—Exercises of this type can be a useful starting place for work on intonation. Dworkin (1991) recommended that these exercises begin with an assessment of the patient's ability to perceive obvious pitch changes in the clinician's voice. If the patient is unable to make these distinctions, the prognosis is poor for improving the patient's pitch control. However, if the patient can tell the difference between the pitch changes, the first step is to have the patient prolong an /a/ at his or her lowest pitch and then at the highest pitch. Once this is established, the patient is asked to sing up and down that pitch range by dividing the range into about eight individual notes. Then the patient is asked to read printed sentences that have arrows written above and below key words indicating the normal pitch changes for those words. For example, an up

arrow at the end of a question would indicate that the patient should raise pitch on the final word; a down arrow at the end of a statement would indicate a decrease in pitch.

- **Intonation profiles**—This task uses lines to show intonation changes in written sentences. Lines immediately below the sentence indicate a flat intonation. Lines above words indicate a rise in pitch. Lines below words indicate a drop in pitch. These lines can be added easily to any written sentence, no matter if it is a statement or question. Of course, for most patients, it is usually best to start with short and simple sentences and then progress to longer sentences. The ultimate goal is to have the patient generalize the pitch changes learned in this structured activity to conversational speech.
- **Chunking utterances into syntactic units**—Duffy (1995) mentioned that some individuals with dysarthria need to learn to divide their utterances into normal pauses within and between sentences. This is necessary because their disorder has limited the number of words they can produce on a single exhalation of air. To compensate for this limitation, this task teaches the patient to inhale at those points in an utterance where there are natural syntactic pauses. Examples of these natural pauses include after introductory clauses or phrases ("In the morning, [inhale] I went shopping at the store."), between clauses or phrases ("She went there, [inhale] but I missed her."), and between short sentences ("I saw the movie. [inhale] It was pretty good."). By inserting their inhalations at points where there are normal pauses in an utterance, individuals with ataxic dysarthria are often able to maintain a more natural rhythm in their speech. This rhythm is lost if inhalations are placed haphazardly within an utterance.

Articulation

Although articulation may improve with a slowed rate of speech, individuals with ataxic dysarthria also may need to concentrate directly on improving their productions of phonemes.

- **Intelligibility Drills**—Intelligibility drills are tasks where the patient is given a list of words or sentences to read and the clinician turns away from the patient so that he or she will only be able to understand the patient's speech if it is articulated clearly. By not looking at the target word list or at the patient's mouth, the clinician will depend on the patient's adequate articulation to understand the target word. If the clinician does not understand the target utterance, the patient needs to determine why the word or words were unclear and then try saying it again. If this second attempt fails, then the clinician can look at the target word and give the patient specific feedback on why he or she could not understand the utterance (e.g., "I didn't know it was *sleep* because I couldn't hear the 'l.' Try it again, and let me really hear the 'l' this time.").

- **Phonetic placement**—In this treatment procedure, the clinician instructs the patient how to correctly position the articulators for a target phoneme before the patient attempts to produce that phoneme in a target word or sentence. Phonetic placement can be valuable in that it educates patients on how certain speech sounds are produced. Many individuals with dysarthria know they are producing speech sounds incorrectly, but they do not understand what has gone wrong. For example, phonetic placement can help speakers with ataxic dysarthria understand why their /d/ sounds like a /z/ or their /v/ sounds like a /b/. This treatment procedure can be useful for increasing awareness of many other articulation errors that can be so puzzling to someone who is unfamiliar with speech production.

- **Exaggerating consonants**—Also known as **overarticulation**, exaggerating consonants is a treatment procedure that teaches the patient to *fully* articulate all consonant phonemes. Darley et al. (1975) suggested that most patients need to concentrate especially on medial and final consonants because these are the sounds most likely to be poorly articulated in connected speech. The improvements in intelligibility can be dramatic when individuals with dysarthria fully articulate the medial and final consonants in words.

- **Minimal contrast drills**—These tasks have the patient concentrate on producing pairs of words that vary by only one phoneme. The distinction between the words can be in the voicing (*park—bark*), manner (*pine—mine*), or place (*sea—she*) of consonants. The distinction also can be between vowels (*man—men*), but usually working on consonants does more to enhance intelligibility in most patients. These word pairs can be used alone, in phrases, or in sentences, depending on the needs of a specific patient.

SUMMARY OF ATAXIC DYSARTHRIA

- Ataxic dysarthria can be caused by any process that results in damage to the cerebellum or the cerebellar control circuits. Degenerative disease and stoke are common causes of ataxic dysarthria.
- Usually, articulation and prosody are affected most significantly in cases of ataxic dysarthria.
- The speech characteristics of ataxic dysarthria include imprecise consonants and irregular articulatory breakdowns.
- Treatment for ataxic dysarthria often concentrates on controlling respiration for speech, increasing articulatory accuracy, and developing optimal rate and intonation in connected speech.

STUDY QUESTIONS

1. Define ataxic dysarthria in your own words.
2. What is the primary function of the cerebellum?
3. Describe the neural pathways leading to and from the cerebellum.
4. What are the two ways that the cerebellum probably influences speech production?
5. What is autosomal dominant cerebellar ataxia of late onset?
6. Describe the three ways in which a tumor can affect cerebellar function.
7. Which two components of speech production are usually affected most in cases of ataxic dysarthria?
8. What is decomposition of movement?
9. Is hypernasality a significant problem in most cases of ataxic dysarthria?
10. Describe an exercise that can help individuals with ataxic dysarthria more accurately control their airflow during speech production.

C H A P T E R

8

Hypokinetic Dysarthria

(continued)

DEFINITIONS OF HYPOKINETIC DYSARTHRIA

Most definitions of hypokinetic dysarthria mention that individuals with this disorder have reduced vocal loudness, a harsh or breathy vocal quality, and abnormal speaking rates. Although these are not all of the characteristics of hypokinetic dysarthria, they are among the most common ones. It is interesting to note that many individuals with this dysarthria have slow speaking rates, but in some there can be an abnormally increased rate of speech. The following two definitions encompass much of the most important aspects of hypokinetic dysarthria.

> Hypokinetic dysarthria is a perceptually distinguishable motor speech disorder associated with basal ganglia control circuit pathology. It may be manifest in any or all of the respiratory, phonatory, resonatory, and articulatory level of speech, but its characteristics are most evident in voice, articulation, and prosody. Its deviant speech characteristics reflect the effects of rigidity, reduced force and range of movement, and slow but sometimes fast repetitive movements on speech. (Duffy, 1995, p. 166)

> Hypokinetic dysarthria [is] characterized by reduced vocal loudness with concomitant harsh-hoarse quality, slow speaking rate with intermittent bursts of rapid fire articulation, excessive and overly long pauses, prolonged syllables, monoloudness, and reduced phonation time. (Dworkin, 1991, p. 9)

NEUROLOGICAL BASIS OF HYPOKINETIC DYSARTHRIA

In several ways, hypokinetic dysarthria is unique. It is the only dysarthria in which increased rate of speech may be one of the symptoms. It also is the only dysarthria in which the vast majority of cases share the same etiological factor (parkinsonism). Because it accounts for so much of the hypokinetic dysarthria seen in clinical caseloads, parkinsonism is considered the de facto cause of this dysarthria throughout most of this chapter. The reader should keep in mind, however, that parkinsonism is not the only cause of hypokinetic dysarthria. A few other disorders can lead to this dysarthria, and they are discussed in the etiology section of this chapter.

Hypokinetic dysarthria occurs when the symptoms of parkinsonism affect the muscles of speech production. The parkinsonian symptoms that have the greatest effect on speech are muscle rigidity, reduced range of motion, and slowed movement. In nearly every instance, these symptoms are caused by dysfunction in the basal ganglia or by damage to the basal ganglia's neural connections to other parts of the CNS. The term *hypokinetic* may be misleading to readers encountering it for the first time. Initially, it may be confused with hypotonia, which is decreased muscle tone. A beginning clinician may consequently assume that an individual with parkinsonism will have weak and floppy muscles. This assumption would be quite wrong, however. Literally, *hypokinetic* means "less motion," not decreased muscle tone. In fact, individuals with parkinsonism usually demonstrate *increased* muscle tone. When applied to individuals with parkinsonism, the term *hypokinetic* describes their decreased range and frequency of movement. For example, individuals with parkinsonism usually demonstrate a shuffling, "baby step" type of walking known as festinating gait, and their ability to express emotion through their facial expressions will be greatly diminished, a phenomenon known as masked facies. In addition, they may blink their eyes infrequently and have difficulty starting or stopping movements. The reasons for these behaviors are discussed in the following paragraphs.

Characteristics of Parkinsonism

The characteristics of parkinsonism are a unique collection of symptoms. One of the most prevalent symptoms is **tremor**. Parkinsonian tremors are seen most commonly in the fingers and hands, but they also can involve the limbs and face. These tremors have a frequency of about 4 to 6 oscillations per second. They are called resting tremors, because they are most noticeable while the body is not moving. Interestingly, the tremors may become less pronounced or disappear completely when the body is completely relaxed or when an affected body part is being moved voluntarily. During moments of agitation or nervousness, however, the tremors may become significantly worse.

Bradykinesia is the slow and reduced range of movement seen in individuals with parkinsonism. It is a very common symptom of parkinsonism. The shuffling walk and the lack of facial expression mentioned previously are good examples of bradykinesia. Limb, trunk, and neck movements also are affected frequently by bradykinesia. Typically, the movements of affected body parts are slow, labored, and very limited in their range. In addition to the difficulties of walking and facial expression, bradykinesia also can affect speech, finger movements, writing, and many other voluntary movements. It is important to note, however, that the slowness and reduced range of movement of bradykinesia is not the result of muscle weakness. Individuals with parkinsonism usually demonstrate nearly normal muscle strength. As with all the symptoms of parkinsonism, bradykinesia is caused by dysfunction in the basal ganglia.

Muscular rigidity is the result of increased muscle tone. The muscles of individuals with this condition are always in a greater than normal state of contraction, both at rest and during movement. Rigidity most typically affects the neck, trunk, and limbs. The effects of rigidity can usually be observed easily. For instance, when an affected body part is pulled to an extended position, there will be constant resistance to the movement. This is sometimes described as "lead pipe resistance," because it feels to the person who is doing the pulling that a piece of soft metal is being bent. In some joints, however, there may be a subtle, rhythmic alteration in the rigidity as a body part is being moved. This intermittent change in rigidity is described as "cogwheel resistance" because of its step-by-step, ratchetlike motion. Although rigidity and bradykinesia are separate symptoms of parkinsonism, rigidity can exacerbate the slowed and restricted movements of bradykinesia.

It should be noted that there are differences between rigidity and spasticity, although they are both the result of increased muscle tone. One of the clearest distinctions between them is how they react to passive movement. In spasticity, there will be an increasing resistance to the passive movement, followed by an abrupt relaxation of the muscle being tested. The increase in resistance is especially evident when the passive movement is rapid. In contrast, patients with rigidity demonstrate a more or less constant resistance to the passive movement, no matter how quickly the examiner moves the affected body part (Wiederholt, 1995).

Akinesia is a delay in the initiation of movements and is yet another common characteristic of parkinsonism. Examples of akinesia can be seen in many of the movements of individuals with parkinsonism. For instance, when an individual with parkinsonism is asked to verbally answer a question, there may be a noticeable pause before any words are spoken. This delayed initiation of speech may last only a few seconds, but sometimes it is much longer. Occasionally, someone with severe akinesia may become "stuck" in a certain posture and be completely unable to move. Strangely, when an individual is stuck in one of these frozen positions, a brief touch from another person is sometimes all that is needed to initiate or continue a movement. In addition to this difficulty in initiating movements, many individuals with parkinsonism can have trouble stopping a movement once it is started. For instance, while reaching for a glass of water, they may knock it over because they were unable to stop reaching once the movement was initiated. Not surprisingly, it is often reported that individuals with akinesia are reluctant to actively move about their home or other surroundings, because they are afraid of being injured when they do so.

Disturbances of postural reflexes also are seen in individuals with parkinsonism. Such disturbances are especially evident when these individuals are doing relatively automatic tasks. For example, they may have difficulty maintaining their balance while walking. In addition, the normal walking arm swing will be absent; their arms will hang stiffly at their sides. If pushed lightly while standing, they are likely to fall, because they cannot quickly shift their center of balance. They may be unable to rise from a chair, because they do not naturally shift their trunk forward as they attempt to stand. Normally, the basal ganglia help regulate these postural reflexes through neural connections with the extrapyramidal system. However, when the basal ganglia are not functioning properly, these postural problems of balance and movement can become obvious.

Although tremor, bradykinesia, rigidity, akinesia, and disturbed postural reflexes are the primary symptoms of parkinsonism, there are numerous other symptoms that may appear in individuals with this disorder. These include depression, swallowing difficulties, dementia, and, of course, hypokinetic dysarthria. Although these additional symptoms do not appear in all individuals with parkinsonism, they can be common features of this disorder nevertheless.

Etiology of Parkinsonism

As already mentioned, parkinsonism is caused by dysfunction in the basal ganglia. The **basal ganglia** are a collection of subcortical, gray matter structures that play an important role in controlling movement

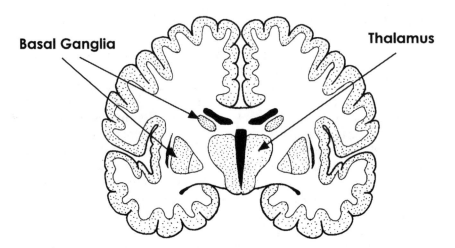

Basal Ganglia

Thalamus

Figure 8–1. Decreased dopamine in the basal ganglia is associated with most causes of parkinsonism. (Adapted from *Neuroscience of Communication*, by D. Webster, 1999. p. 176. San Diego: Singular Publishing Group, Inc. Copyright 1999 by Singular Publishing Group, Inc. Adapted with permission.)

(Figure 8–1). The individual members of the basal ganglia are the caudate nucleus, the globus pallidus, and the putamen. Because the caudate nucleus and the putamen are made of many of the same type of neurons and are functionally related, they are known together as the **striatum**. The basal ganglia are located deep in the brain and are quite complex in their interconnections with each other and with other parts of the CNS. One of the most important neural pathways of the basal ganglia is the looped control circuit that connects it to the cerebral cortex (Figure 8–2). The first part of this control circuit is composed of neural fibers that descend from the cortex. Through these fibers, the cortex transmits information about planned upcoming movements to the basal ganglia. The basal ganglia, in turn, smooth and refine these planned movements, especially movements that are going to be slow and continuous. Once this refinement is completed, the basal ganglia sends the refined neural impulses for the planned movements up to the motor cortex, where they are then transmitted through the pyramidal system to the lower motor neurons and out to the muscles.

To function properly, the basal ganglia depends on the balanced interaction of several neurotransmitters. Two of the most important are dopamine and acetylcholine. Dopamine is largely an inhibitory neurotransmitter and tends to slow neural activity within the striatum. The dopamine used by the striatum is produced by special neurons in the

The Basal Ganglia Control Circuit

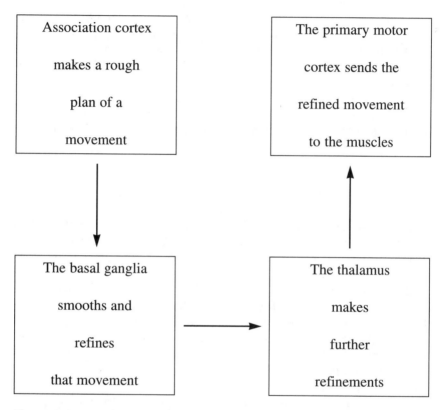

Figure 8–2. A schematic diagram of the basal ganglia control circuit.

substantia nigra, which is a collection of gray matter cells located near the basal ganglia. Acetylcholine also affects the function of the basal ganglia, but unlike dopamine, it has an excitatory effect on these areas of the brain. It tends to facilitate neural firing.

In general, parkinsonism is caused by a reduction of dopamine in the striatum. The loss of dopamine has a profound effect on the workings of the striatum, because it is placed in a state of neurochemical imbalance. When this imbalance occurs, there is relatively too much excitatory neurotransmitter (acetylcholine) acting on the neurons of the striatum compared to the available amount of inhibitory neurotransmitter (dopamine). The higher levels of this excitatory neurotransmitter in the striatum are thereby thought to be the primary cause of the rigidity, bradykinesia, and other symptoms of parkinsonism.

The causes of reduced dopamine in the striatum are varied. In most cases, such as idiopathic Parkinsons disease, the etiology is not understood. In this disease, the dopamine-producing neurons in the substantia nigra slowly begin to degenerate for unknown reasons. As they degenerate, they produce less and less dopamine for use in the striatum, which then is unable to function properly. There are numerous other ways in which these dopamine-producing neurons can be damaged, including the effects of drugs and toxic poisoning, damage from infections, tumors, head injury, cerebral anoxia, and cerebrovascular disease.

Pharmacological Treatments for Parkinsonism

There are several pharmacological treatments for hypokinetic movement disorders. One treatment approach is to replace dopamine in the striatum. However, direct dosages of dopamine are not effective because they cannot pass the blood-brain barrier and, consequently, will not reach the striatum. (The blood-brain barrier is the body's mechanism that controls the flow of matter from the blood stream to the extracellular fluid in the brain. Part of this barrier's effectiveness is the tight arrangement of the cells in the walls of the cerebral capillaries.) Because of the blood-brain barrier, dopamine replacement treatments use a precursor of dopamine known as l-dopa, a chemical that can reach the striatum and then is converted into dopamine by the brain. Once in the striatum, this drug compensates for the dopamine that is not being produced by the substantia nigra.

Another treatment approach attempts to correct the neurotransmitter imbalance in the basal ganglia by decreasing the amount of acetylcholine activity in the striatum. Anticholinergic drugs act to either deplete acetylcholine in the basal ganglia or to interfere with its effect on these brain structures. In some individuals with parkinsonism, the best treatment results occur when l-dopa combined with certain anticholinergic drugs.

The effectiveness of these treatments is well established. l-dopa can significantly reduce tremor, bradykinesia, akinesia, and rigidity in many hypokinetic movement disorders. In addition, l-dopa treatment can prolong the life of an individual if it is started early enough in the course of some disorders. Although l-dopa is effective on many symptoms of hypokinetic disorders, Wiederholt (1995) reported that the speech disturbances associated with these disorders are least helped by this drug. In addition, the side effects of l-dopa can range from minor to quite serious. The minor problems include gastrointestinal disturbance, poor control of blood pressure, insomnia, and agitation. The more serious side effects usually appear after a prolonged course of treatment and include such significant psychiatric symptoms as hallucinations, severe agitation, decreased social inhibitions, and paranoid delusions. Prolonged treatments with l-dopa also can cause abnormal involuntary movements (choreiform movements) of the limbs, head and neck, and orofacial muscles.

Anticholinergic drugs also may reduce the major symptoms of many hypokinetic movement disorders, but their negative effects can be just as significant as those in l-dopa treatment. The minor side effects include such problems as dry mouth, dizziness, dilated pupils, and clumsiness. The more serious side effects include inappropriate emotional outbursts, delusions, hallucinations, and confusion.

Unfortunately, none of the pharmacological treatments for hypokinetic movement disorders are cures. They can reduce many of the symptoms and can slow the progression of some degenerative disorders, but they are not permanent cures. They do not return an affected individual to completely normal motor functions. In fact, these drugs eventually become ineffective in treating progressive hypokinetic disorders.

ETIOLOGIES OF HYPOKINETIC DYSARTHRIA

Parkinsonism is a collective term for a group of different disorders that share many of the same symptoms. It is sometimes used interchangeably with the term Parkinson syndrome. In general, the shared symptoms of parkinsonism are those which were discussed previously: tremor, bradykinesia, muscle rigidity, akinesia, and disturbed postural reflexes. In the following section of this chapter, the major causes of hypokinetic dysarthria are examined, starting with three disorders that are classed under parkinsonism.

Idiopathic Parkinson's Disease

Idiopathic Parkinson's disease is the most common form of parkinsonism and is the single most frequent cause of hypokinetic dysarthria.

This disease is the result of the progressive degeneration of dopamine producing neurons in the substantia nigra. As mentioned previously, the reason why these neurons degenerate is unknown, hence the label "idiopathic." It affects about 20 individuals per 100,000 each year, with males and females being affected equally. It usually occurs in individuals between the ages of 40 and 70 years and typically follows a slowly progressive course that lasts for years. The first signs of Parkinson's disease often include restlessness, rapid tiredness, and such sensory signs as coldness, numbness, or tingling. Duffy (1995) noted that hypokinetic dysarthria also can be one of the first symptoms of this disease. As the disease progresses, these early signs are joined by the major symptoms of tremor, rigidity, and so forth. In about 50% to 75% of cases, l-dopa treatments are successful in treating most of the major symptoms. However, as discussed, these treatments can reduce the severity of the symptoms, but they do not stop the progression of the disorder.

Additional symptoms of this disorder include dementia, which is present in 8% to 30% of cases. In most cases, it is difficult to determine if this dementia is caused only by the Parkinson's disease or by an accompanying occurrence of Alzheimer disease. Significant depression also has been reported in as many as 50% of patients. Warlow (1991) reported that most individuals with Parkinson's disease are ultimately confined to bed and die of pneumonia, urinary tract infections, or septicemia (the persistent presence of toxic microorganisms in the blood, commonly called blood poisoning).

Neuroleptic-Induced Parkinsonism

Neuroleptic-induced parkinsonism is the second most common form of parkinsonism. It is a condition that is a negative side effect of using antipsychotic (neuroleptic) drugs. These drugs can be very successful in treating the confusion and agitation in psychotic patients, but their long-term use can result in this form of parkinsonism. The neuroleptic drugs that have this side effect include chlorpromazine, trifluoperazine, and prochlorperazine. The appearance of parkinsonian symptoms depends on the drug and the dosage levels. For example, about 90% of patients taking trifluoperazine may show subtle, variable signs of tremor, rigidity, and, in particular, bradykinesia. It usually takes about 2 to 4 weeks of taking the drug before these parkinsonian symptoms appear. It is not clearly understood how neuroleptic drugs cause the symptoms of parkinsonism. It is known, however, that some of these drugs increase the amount of acetylcholine in the basal ganglia. Consequently, it is supposed that this increase in acetylcholine results in relatively lower levels of dopamine in the basal ganglia and thereby causes the parkinsonian symptoms.

The signs of neuroleptic-induced parkinsonism usually disappear within weeks of discontinuing use of the drugs. However, stopping the drug treatment is often not an option for many of these individuals, because their psychosis will return. In these cases, the individual will continue to take the neuroleptic medication, but they also will take additional medications to treat their parkinsonian symptoms. Interestingly, l-dopa cannot be used to treat the hypokinetic movement disorders in these individuals because it tends to increase their psychotic symptoms.

Postencephalitic Parkinsonism

Postencephalitic parkinsonism is caused by viral encephalitis. It is a relatively common disorder, and, unlike idiopathic Parkinson's disease, it can affect children. In postencephalitic parkinsonism, the effects of the infection are concentrated in the basal ganglia, which consequently results in decreased amounts of dopamine in this area of the brain. The parkinsonian symptoms appear several weeks or months after the acute stage of the infection. In the majority of cases, these symptoms are identical to those in idiopathic Parkinson's disease. In some instances, the initial symptoms of the infection are so mild that they are unrecognized. Nevertheless, the basal ganglia is still damaged and the result can be parkinsonism. Certain cognitive deficits are associated with children who develop postencephalitic parkinsonism, including increased distractibility and impaired abstract reasoning. Pharmacological treatment of this disorder is the same as for idiopathic Parkinson's disease, usually l-dopa therapy.

Traumatic Head Injury

Head trauma can selectively damage the substantia nigra or basal ganglia. The trauma can be either a single event or repeated injuries over time. Duffy (1995) noted that the cumulative effects of repeated blows to the head, such as what occurs in boxing, can damage the substantia nigra and may result in **punch drunk encephalopathy**, a disorder characterized by memory deficits, slowed movements, and dysarthria.

Cerebral anoxia also has been known to selectively affect the basal ganglia to a greater degree than other areas of the brain, although the exact reason for this is unknown. In such cases, bradykinesia and rigidity may appear days or weeks after the patient returns to consciousness. Co-occurring cognitive and pyramidal system deficits probably will be present as well.

Toxic Metal Poisoning

An often-cited cause of parkinsonian symptoms is long-term exposure to manganese, a metal used in the manufacturing of iron, aluminum, and copper alloys. The early signs of manganese poisoning, which occurs most often in miners, include irritability, insomnia, and emotional outbursts. Dementia usually co-occurs with the parkinsonian signs in the later stages of chronic exposure to this metal.

Stroke

Although references are sometimes made to "arteriosclerotic parkinsonism" or "vascular parkinsonism," Wiederholt (1995) stated that there is no credible evidence for such a diagnostic classification. Nevertheless, it has been documented that a single stroke can affect the basal ganglia and cause the sudden onset of parkinsonian symptoms, although it certainly is rare. Warlow (1991) indicated that such a stroke results in parkinsonian symptoms on the side of the body opposite to the lesion, with a majority of cases showing spontaneous improvement over time. Compared to a single stroke resulting in parkinsonism, it is more likely that parkinsonism symptoms will appear in an individual who has suffered multiple strokes. In instances such as these, there will probably be numerous associated disorders, including other motor system deficits, visuospatial impairments, and speech and language problems.

SPEECH CHARACTERISTICS OF HYPOKINETIC DYSARTHRIA

The speech of individuals with hypokinetic dysarthria is usually quite distinctive. Errors of prosody and articulation are the most noticeable speech characteristic in this type of dysarthria. Overall, individuals with hypokinetic dysarthria give the impression that the sequencing and placement of their articulatory movements are fairly accurate, but the range of these movements is greatly restricted. It is as if their speech movements are compressed and abbreviated. As is discussed in the following paragraphs, most of the speech characteristics of hypokinetic dysarthria are a result of bradykinesia (reduced range and speed of movement), akinesia (delays in the initiation of movement), and muscle rigidity. In the most severe cases, the tremors so commonly associated with parkinsonism also can affect the speech musculature, resulting in tremulous phonations.

Prosody

Darley et al. (1969a, 1969b) found that **monopitch**, **reduced stress**, and **monoloudness** were the three most prominent speech characteristics of hypokinetic dysarthria (see Table 8–1). They attributed these prosodic errors to a limited range of motion in the laryngeal musculature and to a lack of "vigor" in the contractions of these muscles. These prosodic errors are most evident in verbal tasks that normally include variations in pitch and loudness, such as conversational speech, reading sentences or paragraphs, and trying to verbally convey emotions.

Table 8–1. The Most Common Speech Production Errors in 32 Individuals With Hypokinetic Dysarthria

Rank	Speech Production Errors
1	Monopitch
2	Reduced stress
3	Monoloudness
4	Imprecise consonants
5	Inappropriate silences
6	Short rushes
7	Harsh voice quality
8	Breathy voice (continuous)
9	Pitch level
10	Variable rate

Source: From "Clusters of Diagnostic Patterns of Dysarthria," by F. L. Darley, A. E. Aronson, and J. R. Brown, 1969, *Journal of Speech and Hearing Research, 12*, p. 258. Copyright 1969 by American Speech-Language-Hearing Association. Reprinted with permission.

Darley et al. also noted **inappropriate silences** in the speech of their subjects. These silent pauses are probably the result of the akinesia, which makes it difficult for affected individuals to initiate a motor response. Clinical observations suggest that these moments of silence appear most frequently at the beginning of an spoken sentence or between sentences. They often may last for only 2 or 3 s, but longer lapses can occur. When combined with the condition's typical expressionless facial movements, these silent moments sometimes mislead beginning clinicians into assuming the patient did not hear a question or perhaps has lost his or her train of thought.

Several speech rate abnormalities also can be present in hypokinetic dysarthria. An overall **increased rate of speech** is the most notable of these. Although most individuals with hypokinetic dysarthria do not demonstrate a consistently increased speech rate, it has been seen in some cases. It has been suggested that increased speech rate is related to the difficulties some individuals with parkinsonism have in stopping a voluntary movement once it is started (Hirose, 1986). If severe enough, this increased rate of speech can result in the "blurred" articulation of phonemes. Of course, this can contribute to the imprecise production of consonants, which will be discussed presently. **Short rushes of speech** are probably more common in hypokinetic dysarthria than a constant increase in speech rate. When these short rushes occur, they may have a stop-and-go quality, with a brief pause being followed immediately by the quick production of several words. Darley et al. (1969a, 1969b) found these short rushes of speech to be the sixth most common characteristic of hypokinetic dysarthria, appearing in 19 of their 32 subjects. Finally, it must be noted that some studies have found cases of decreased rate of speech in individuals with this dysarthria (Ludlow, Connor, & Bassich, 1987). It would appear, therefore, that there can be significant individual differences in speech rate abnormalities in cases of hypokinetic dysarthria, ranging from slow to fast.

Articulation

There can be numerous types of articulation errors in hypokinetic dysarthria. According to Darley et al. (1969a, 1969b), one of the most common is **imprecise consonants**. In many cases, the imprecise production of consonants is caused by reduced range of movement by the articulators, which consequently results in distorted and incorrect productions of phonemes. For instance, stop consonants can sound very much like fricatives, because the articulators are unable to completely block the airflow. Fricative consonants can have a distorted "mushy" quality, because the point of airflow constriction is slightly larger than what is needed for normal articulation. Affricate consonants can reflect a combination of these errors, because they contain both a stop phase and a fricativelike release phase. These types of errors in the production of consonants are sometimes described as articulatory undershoot (Duffy, 1995).

Two unusual dysfluencies also have been noted in the speech of individuals with hypokinetic dysarthria. The first of these is **repeated phonemes**. Duffy (1995) indicated that these repetitions usually take place at the beginning of an utterance or after a pause. They are often very quick and may be produced with very limited movement of the articulators. In fact, they can sound like a prolonged vowel because of how rapidly they are produced. The other type of dysfluency is **palilalia**, which is the compulsive, increasingly rapid repetition of a word or phrase. Although it was not noted in any of the subjects studied by Darley et al. (1969a, 1969b), palilalia may be present in some individuals with parkinsonism. This phenomenon may be most clearly evident to a listener when the affected individual makes a single-word utterance, perhaps in answer to a yes-no question. The response, for example, will be the repetition of "yes, yes, yes, yes, yes, yes" with a quickly increasing rate of speech until the utterance fades into a soft, blurred mumble. Both of these dysfluencies may be neurologically related to the festinating gait of individuals with parkinsonism, in which they sometimes cannot stop themselves from walking past their destination. In a very similar manner, some hypokinetic speakers may not be able to stop saying a syllable or word once they have started an utterance.

Phonation

A **harsh** or **breathy voice quality** is common in most individuals with hypokinetic dysarthria, although these may not be the most noticeable speech errors in this disorder. Logemann, Fisher, Boshes, and Blonsky (1978) found that 89% of their 200 subjects with Parkinsons disease had vocal qualities that were breathy, hoarse, rough, or tremulous. This finding indicates how widespread these errors of phonation can be in this dysarthria. Darley et al. (1969a, 1969b) also noted phonatory deficits in their subjects but ranked them in the bottom half of the most prominent speech errors in hypokinetic dysarthria. They described these errors as either a harsh or breathy voice quality and ranked them, respectively, as the seventh and eighth most prominent speech characteristics of their 32 subjects with parkinsonism.

Several studies provide evidence that the harsh or breathy vocal quality of hypokinetic dysarthria is caused by incomplete vocal fold closure during phonation (Cisler, 1927, as cited in Darley et al., 1975; Lehiste, 1965). When the vocal folds fail to completely close during phonation, air leaks through the partly open glottis and causes an audibly turbulent noise. In the more severe cases, vocal quality may become so breathy as to be more of a whisper. When combined with decreased loudness (discussed shortly), this whispering vocal quality often makes the individual's speech unintelligible. Duffy (1995) stated, "In general, dysphonia can be the presenting, most prominent and debilitating speech feature in people with hypokinetic dysarthria" (p. 175). In addition to this whispered dysphonia, moments of aphonia (complete loss of phonation) also may occur in connected speech, even in the less severely involved individuals.

Low pitch can be another phonatory characteristic of hypokinetic dysarthria. Darley et al. (1969a, 1969b) rated it as the ninth most prominent speech error in their subjects with hypokinetic dysarthria. However, other studies have found increased pitch in hypokinetic speakers (Canter, 1963; Ludlow & Bassich, 1984). Taken as a whole, these studies suggest that patients with hypokinetic dysarthria can have significant individual-to-individual differences in pitch.

Respiration

Respiratory difficulties have been noted in some individuals with hypokinetic dysarthria. For example, it has been observed that these individuals may have breathing rates that are faster than normal. It also has been noted that these individuals frequently have paradoxical movements of the muscles of exhalation and inhalation, which means that the respiratory muscles of the chest and the diaphragm are not coordinated during breathing. Last, many individuals with hypokinetic dysarthria have reduced range of movement in their respiratory muscles. These respiratory problems result in shallow breath support, poorly controlled exhalations of air for speech, and short breathing cycles. Each of these factors can contribute to many of the speech errors in hypokinetic dysarthria. The rapid, short breathing cycles, for instance, may be a partial cause of the short rushes of speech discussed previously. The shallow breath support may make a significant contribution to the breathy, soft phonations of this dysarthria.

Resonance

Although hypernasality can be present in some cases of hypokinetic dysarthria, its severity is usually mild. Most individuals with this dysarthria do not demonstrate significant deficits of resonance. For instance, Logemann et al. (1978) found mild hypernasality in only 10% of their subjects with Parkinson's disease.

KEY EVALUATION TASKS FOR HYPOKINETIC DYSARTHRIA

Duffy (1995) recommended three key evaluation tasks to help highlight the speech errors commonly heard in hypokinetic dysarthria:

1. Conversational speech and reading are useful for evoking the many errors of prosody that may be present in this dysarthria. These errors include monopitch, reduced stress, monoloudness, and inappropriate silences. Connected speech samples also can be useful in detecting if short rushes of speech are present. This is heard when several words of a longer utterance are said hurriedly together, first preceded by and then followed by a brief pause.
2. Speech AMRs can highlight articulation errors, including imprecise consonant productions, variable rates of articulation, and the blurring of syllables.
3. Vowel prolongations can be helpful in assessing vocal quality.
4. Conversational speech, AMRs, and vowel prolongation also can be used to detect other characteristics of hypokinetic dysarthria, such as decreased loudness, low pitch, and repeated phonemes.

TREATMENT OF HYPOKINETIC DYSARTHRIA

The most widely used treatment for the underlying pathologies that cause hypokinetic dysarthria is pharmacological, usually the administration of drugs based on l-dopa. Most patients treated with l-dopa or anticholinergic drugs show some improvements in their bradykinesia, rigidity, and tremor (Warlow, 1991). Although hypokinetic dysarthria may not respond as well to these drugs as do the other motor disturbances associated with parkinsonism, there often are some improvements in speech production nevertheless. Although the drugs can have some positive effects on the speech deficits in parkinsonism, behaviorally and instrumentally based tasks are an important part of the clinical treatment plan. There are numerous procedures that speech-language pathologists can use to help these patients communicate more effectively.

Articulation

The most common articulation deficit in hypokinetic dysarthria is imprecise consonant production, which is sometimes described as giving the patient's speech a "mushy" quality. As previously mentioned, this problem is often the result of reduced range of motion in the articulators. This deficit can be compounded by the increased rate of speech that occurs in some patients with parkinsonism. The articulation errors in hypokinetic dysarthria can be treated in several ways. In general, the treatments are divided into rate reduction, stretching, and traditional articulation tasks.

Rate Reduction

In many individuals with hypokinetic dysarthria, slowing the rate of speech can improve articulation, because it allows the articulators more time to reach the target positions needed to accurately produce phonemes. The slower rate also gives the listener more time to process what is being spoken. Prosody also may appear more natural when rate is slowed. A number of different rate control procedures have been used to slow the speech of individuals with hypokinetic dysarthria.

- **Pacing boards**—These are devices with finger-width slots along their length (Figure 8–3). Using pacing boards is simple. The patient is instructed to place a finger in the first slot and begin reading or repeating a short sentence, and each time a word is spoken move the finger to the next slot. That is, the patient should only say one word every time the finger is moved to the next slot on the board. By slowing their rate of speech, this procedure can produce noticeable improvements in intelligibility in many individuals with hypokinetic dysarthria. One of the drawbacks of a pacing board can be the patient's reluctance to use it in public when speaking to

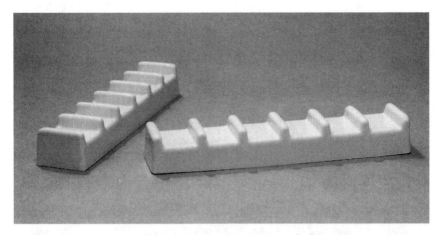

Figure 8–3. Inexpensive plastic pacing boards, which may be useful in slowing the rate of speech in some individuals with hypokinetic dysarthria.

strangers. As a consequence, pacing boards are often used only in the home, although they are very portable and are used successfully in public by some individuals with this dysarthria.

- **Hand or finger tapping**—In the beginning of this task, the clinician sets the pace for repeating or reading sentences by tapping his or her hand or finger. The patient attempts to speak one syllable for each of the clinician's taps. Once this rate is established, the patient does the tapping to control the rate of speech production. One problem with this procedure is that many individuals with parkinsonism have difficulty maintaining a slow, steady rate as they tap. As a result, their tapping will increase along with their rate of speech. Pacing boards seem to be a good option for patients who show this problem. The requirement of having to move their finger up and over to the next slot tends to keep their rate of speech steadier than only using hand or finger tapping to set the rate.
- **Alphabet boards**—Another way to slow the rate of someone with this dysarthria is the use of an alphabet board (Figure 8–4). This is simply a piece of paper with all of the letters of the alphabet printed in large, dark print. The numbers 1 to 10 also may be printed on it. The patient is told to use the board by pointing to the first letter of every word as it is being spoken. This procedure can increase intelligibility in two ways. It slows

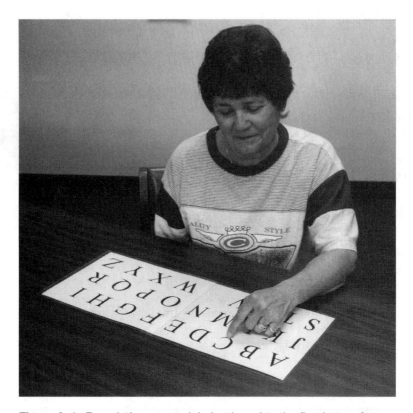

Figure 8–4. By pointing on an alphabet board to the first letter of every word they speak, individuals with hypokinetic dysarthria are forced to slow their rate of speech. The listener also receives a first letter visual cue of the target word, which often facilitates comprehension.

the patient's speech and allows for better articulatory contact. It also gives the listener a visual cue as to what word is being spoken. As with pacing boards, the use of an alphabet board can have an immediate effect on intelligibility. There are drawbacks, however. Many patients will be reluctant to use this procedure in public, which may limit its use to the home. In addition, individuals with hypokinetic dysarthria with even mild dementia may find this procedure beyond their cognitive capabilities.

• **Delayed auditory feedback**—This electronic device "feeds" patients their own voice after a short delay, usually of approximately 50 to 150 ms (Figure 8–5). To maintain fluent speech

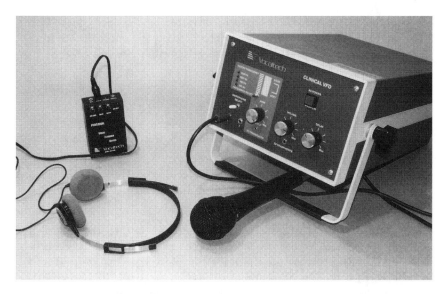

Figure 8–5. Two delayed auditory feedback instruments.

while listening to their own delayed speech, most patients must slow their rate of speaking. Although used frequently to slow the speaking rate of people who stutter, delayed auditory feedback also has been used to slow the rate of speech in individuals with hypokinetic dysarthria. The effectiveness of this procedure to slow the rate of speech and increase intelligibility has been demonstrated in some studies (Adams, 1994; Yorkston et al., 1988) but not in others (Dagenais, Southwood, & Lee, 1998). Downie, Low, and Lindsay (1981) found that delayed auditory feedback was effective in 2 of their 11 subjects with parkinsonism. Because of these mixed results, it may be useful to attempt a short trial period of delayed auditory feedback treatment to determine if it is effective in reducing a given patient's rate of speech.

- **Reciting syllables to a metronome**—Dworkin (1991) suggested using a metronome to set the pace of syllable production. In this task, the metronome is set to the appropriate rate, and the patient is asked to recite or read familiar passages such as the Pledge of Allegiance, a well-known poem, and so forth. The patient should produce one syllable for every beat of the metronome. Although the resulting speech will sound automated, this is acceptable because the goal is to build the patient's awareness of a more appropriate speech rate. With enough practice, the slower pace set by the metronome may become habituated into the patient's conversational speech.

Stretching Exercises

The stretching exercises discussed in the following paragraphs are very similar to those used in treating spastic dysarthria. These tasks are designed to reduce the increased muscle tone of the articulators and increase the range of motion in these same structures.

- **Tongue stretching exercises**—Dworkin (1991) described a series of passive tongue stretching exercises in which the clinician gently grasps the patient's tongue with a gauze pad and carefully pulls it outward until resistance is felt. This protruded position is held for 10 s. The next steps have the clinician gently pulling the protruded tongue to the left or right sides of the mouth and again holding the position for 10 s. Dworkin cautioned against pulling the tongue too forcefully and encouraged the clinician and patient to have patience during these tasks. Active tongue stretching movements by the patient also can be used to increase the range and accuracy of tongue movements (Duffy, 1995; Swigert, 1997). Examples of these exercises include having the patient protrude the tongue fully, elevating the tongue tip toward the nose, lowering the tongue tip toward the chin, and holding the tongue at the corners of the mouth. Other active tongue stretching exercises include elevating the back of the tongue to the soft palate and pressing the tongue tip into the cheek. *Although these active tongue stretching movements have the benefit of promoting increased strength, they also may increase hypertonicity in some patients.* The clinician should monitor changes in muscle tone carefully. If the active stretching exercises prove to be counterproductive, the passive stretching exercises should be used exclusively.
- **Lip stretching exercises**—In passive lip stretching exercises, the clinician grasps one of the lips gently with a gauze pad and carefully pulls it out and away from the face, holding the position for about 10 s. Active lip stretching tasks have the patient making the movements. They include holding a smile, pursing the lips, and puffing out the cheeks. Again, the clinician should

monitor any changes in lip muscle tone when active stretching exercises have been recommended. If increased muscle tone is noted, passive exercises should be used exclusively.

- **Jaw stretching exercises**—Swigert (1997) recommended two stretching exercises to lessen rigidity in the jaw muscles. First, the patient attempts to hold a maximum opening of the jaw, both with and without physical assistance from the clinician. Then the patient attempts to hold the jaw lateralized first to the right and then to the left, both with and without physical assistance from the clinician. The clinician determines the length of time the patient is required to hold the position and the number of repetitions that should be completed during this task.

Traditional Articulation Treatments

Traditional articulation treatments also are recommended for the imprecise consonant productions in patients with hypokinetic dysarthria. These tasks concentrate on increasing the patient's awareness of articulation errors and practicing optimal phoneme productions.

- **Intelligibility Drills**—Intelligibility drills are tasks in which the patient is given a list of words or sentences to read aloud. The clinician then turns away from the patient so that he or she will only be able to understand the patient's speech if it is articulated clearly. By not looking at the target word list or at the patient's mouth, the clinician will depend entirely on the patient's adequate articulation to understand a target word. If the clinician does not understand the target utterance, the patient needs to determine why the word or words were unclear and then try saying it again. If this second attempt fails, the clinician can look at the target word and give the patient specific feedback on why the utterance was not understood (e.g., "I didn't know it was *sleep* because I couldn't hear the *l*. Try it again, and let me really hear the *l* this time.").
- **Phonetic placement**—In this procedure, the clinician instructs the patient on the correct position of the articulators before an attempt is made to produce a target sound. Phonetic placement can be valuable, in that it educates patients on how certain speech sounds are produced. Many affected individuals know they are producing speech sounds incorrectly, but they do not have much understanding of why their productions are in error. For instance, phonetic placement can be helpful in edu-

cating individuals with hypokinetic dysarthria why their production of /d/ sounds like a /z/. This procedure can be helpful in explaining many additional articulation errors that may be puzzling to someone who is unfamiliar with speech production.

- **Exaggerating consonants**—Also known as **overarticulation**, exaggerating consonants is a treatment procedure that teaches the patient to *fully* articulate all consonant phonemes. Darley et al. (1975) suggested that most patients need to concentrate especially on medial and final consonants because these are the sounds most likely to be poorly articulated in connected speech. The improvements in intelligibility can be dramatic when individuals with dysarthria fully articulate the medial and final consonants in words.

- **Minimal contrast drills**—These tasks have the patient concentrate on producing pairs of words that vary by only one phoneme. The distinction between the words can be in the voicing (*park—bark*), manner (*pine—mine*), or place (*sea—she*) of consonants. The distinction also can be between vowels (*man—men*), but usually working on consonants does more to enhance intelligibility in most patients. These word pairs can be used alone, in phrases, or in sentences, depending on the needs of each specific patient.

Phonation

Because many individuals with hypokinetic dysarthria only partially adduct their vocal folds, they may have a harsh or breathy vocal quality when speaking. When this abnormal vocal quality is combined with poor respiratory support, their speech also may have significantly reduced loudness. Most of the following treatment tasks are the same as those used for flaccid dysarthria. These activities are designed to increase phonatory effort so as to bring the vocal folds together in a more fully adducted position.

- **Pushing and pulling procedures**—Sometimes described as **effortful closure techniques**, pushing and pulling procedures help the vocal folds adduct by providing an overall increase in muscle contractions in the torso and neck. In contrast to cases of flaccid dysarthria in which these procedures are used to increase strength in the laryngeal muscles, they are used in hypokinetic dysarthria to overcome reduced range of motion in the laryngeal muscles. One example of these techniques is having a sitting patient push up on the arms of a chair while phonating an /a/. Another example would be to have the patient pull up on the edge of a heavy table while phonating.

- **Hard glottal attack**—Some patients can phonate better when they begin an utterance with a hard glottal attack. Dworkin (1991) described a complete exercise for this procedure. The basic steps are to have the patient hold a deep breath, bear down, and attempt to phonate a tight /a/. This tight phonation should be modified into a more normal vocal quality as soon as possible to avoid the adverse side effects of repeated hard glottal attacks during speech.

- **Voice amplifiers**—A small, portable voice amplifier can be a useful tool for individuals whose voice quality is breathy and soft. These devices have a detachable microphone that the patient speaks into and a speaker that amplifies the voice. A volume knob controls the output from the amplifier. Although these devices are simple to use, some training usually is needed to help the patient determine how far to hold the microphone from the mouth and how to adjust the volume knob. These devices can be quite helpful for some patients. As a trial, the author once recommended a voice amplifier for a patient with Parkinson's disease whose voice was very soft. Ironically, his wife was very hard of hearing. Once they learned how to use the device, the two of them were so pleased with its performance that they were no longer interested in continuing the regular treatment sessions. One wishes all dismissals from treatment were so satisfactory.

- **Instrumental biofeedback**—Numerous electric devices can provide visual or auditory feedback on pitch, loudness, and rate of speech. One example of this type of instrument is the Vocalite, a small device that contains a light and an internal microphone. When a patient's vocal loudness reaches a certain intensity, the light will shine until the loudness falls below a predetermined level. As long as the patient's speech loudness remains above that predetermined level, the light will remain on. The Vocalite's intensity level is adjustable to meet the specific needs of each patient. Another biofeedback device is the Visi-Pitch. This computerized instrument gives patients a real-time visual display of their pitch and loudness while they are speaking. By watching a graphic display on the Visi-Pitch screen, patients are able to adjust their pitch or loudness to reach desired levels of performance.

Several studies have documented the effectiveness of instrumental biofeedback devices to enhance the speech of individuals with hypokinetic dysarthria (Johnson & Pring, 1990; Rubow & Swift, 1985; Scott & Caird, 1983). Although initial treatment gains can be achieved with these devices, it should not be assumed that using them ensures the successful transfer of these gains to outside settings. Rubow and Swift (1985) found that their subject's in-clinic improvements in speech loudness did not carryover to nonclinic locations. Naturally, such difficulties with carryover are not just a problem in the treatment of hypokinetic dysarthria with instrumental biofeedback. They are common to the treatment of all speech and language deficits.

Respiration

The shallow breath support that can occur in hypokinetic dysarthria may cause shortened phrases and decreased loudness in the speech of affected individuals. In addition, it can contribute to the breathy quality of their phonation. The respiratory treatments for hypokinetic dysarthria are many of the same used in the treatment of flaccid dysarthria.

- **Speak immediately on exhalation**—Because of their shallow breath support, many patients with hypokinetic dysarthria have very limited amounts of subglottic air. By cueing the patients to begin phonating immediately on exhalation, they can use more of their available air for speech. Swigert (1997) suggested that the first step in this exercise is to have the patients place a hand on the abdomen and begin a simple /m/ phonation the moment the hand starts to move inward on the exhalation. The clinician can place his or her hand on the patient's hand to know when to cue the patient to begin the phonation, if necessary.
- **Cues to inhale completely**—Sometimes breath support for speech can be increased by reminding the patient to inhale fully before speaking. The clinician will probably need to give frequent reminders about this early in treatment. The goal is to have this deeper inhalation become a habitual part of conversational speech. If it does not overwhelm the patient with too much information, it is often effective to combine the cues to inhale completely with reminders to speak immediately on exhalation.
- **Slow and controlled exhalation**—In this simple task, the patient is asked to inhale fully and then exhale in a slow, steady

stream. Using a stopwatch, the clinician times the length of the exhalation. The goal is to increase the length and steadiness of the air flow over several sessions. Dworkin (1991) described an advanced variation on this task in which the patient is asked to inhale fully, begin a slow exhalation for 3 s, stop the exhalation by holding the breath for about 1 s, then continuing with the exhalation. The difficulty can be increased until the patient is holding and releasing the air three times on a single breath.

- **Stop phonation early**—Because of paradoxical respiratory muscle movements, individuals with hypokinetic dysarthria often demonstrate shallow respiration. As is typical for individuals with this difficulty, they may try to phonate for a longer period than their limited subglottic air supply allows. This results in speaking on residual air, which can cause a harsh vocal quality, decreased loudness, and an increased rate of speech. Consequently, it is often necessary for a patient to learn to stop an utterance before running low on air. This can often be accomplished initially by the clinician providing verbal and visual cues that tell the patient when to stop phonating and take another breath. Over time the cues can be faded as the patient become more independent at stopping phonation before speaking on residual air.

- **Optimal breath group**—This task is similar to the stopping phonation early procedure. The optimal breath group task teaches the patient how many syllables or words can be said clearly on one full inhalation (Linebaugh, 1983). Once a baseline has been established, the patient can work on increasing the length of the breath group, perhaps through deeper inhalations, more controlled exhalations, or beginning phonations immediately on exhalation.

Prosody

As already mentioned, prosody often can be improved by slowing the rate of speech in individuals with hypokinetic dysarthria. The following paragraphs describe some of the other procedures recommended for making the prosody of these speakers appear more natural.

- **Intonation profiles**—This task uses lines to show intonation changes in written sentences. Lines immediately below a sentence indicate a flat intonation. Lines above words indicate a rise in pitch. Lines below words indicate a drop in pitch. These lines can be added easily to any written sentence, no matter if it is a statement or question. Of course, for most patients, it is usually best to start with short and simple sentences and then progress to longer sentences. The ultimate goal is to have the patient generalize the pitch changes learned in this structured activity to conversational speech.

- **Contrastive stress drills**—These tasks are usually designed so that the clinician asks a question, and the patient answers it by adding stress on key words to convey the intended meaning of the answer. For example, the clinician may ask the following question about a picture of a man playing football, "Is the man playing basketball?" The patient will answer, "No. The man is playing *football*." The clinician's next question might be, "Is the woman playing football?" The patient's answer to this question would be, "No, the *man* is playing football." The length of the questions and the complexity of the pictures for this task can easily be varied according to the abilities of each patient.

- **Chunking utterances into syntactic units**—Duffy (1995) mentioned that some individuals with dysarthria need to learn to divide their utterances according to normal pauses within and between sentences. This is necessary, because their disorder has limited the number of words they can produce on a single exhalation of air. To compensate for this limitation, this task teaches the patient to inhale at those points in an utterance where there are natural syntactic pauses. Examples of these natural pauses include after introductory clauses or phrases ("In the morning, [inhale] I went shopping at the store."), between clauses or phrases ("She went there, [inhale] but I missed her."), and between short sentences ("I saw the movie. [inhale] It was pretty good."). By inserting their inhalations at points where there are normal pauses in an utterance, individuals with hypokinetic dysarthria are often able to maintain a more natural rhythm in their speech. This rhythm is lost if inhalations are placed haphazardly within an utterance.

SUMMARY OF HYPOKINETIC DYSARTHRIA

- Any process that damages the basal ganglia can cause hypokinetic dysarthria. This dysarthria is closely associated with parkinsonism, which is a collective term that includes such disorders as idiopathic Parkinson disease and drug-induced parkinsonism.

- The symptoms of parkinsonism are tremor, bradykinesia, muscular rigidity, akinesia, and disturbances of postural reflexes.
- The most common cause of hypokinetic dysarthria is idiopathic Parkinson's disease. This disease is caused by decreased amounts of the neurotransmitter dopamine in the portion of the basal ganglia called the striatum.
- The speech characteristics of hypokinetic dysarthria include harsh vocal quality, reduced stress, monoloudness, and imprecise consonants.
- Treatment of hypokinetic dysarthria should concentrate on improving articulatory precision, increasing phonatory effort, and promoting more natural prosody. Individuals with increased rate of speech can often benefit from rate control tasks.

STUDY QUESTIONS

1. Define hypokinetic dysarthria in your own words.
2. What are the characteristic symptoms of parkinsonism?
3. Describe how the substantia nigra and the striatum are involved in the cause of parkinsonism.
4. What is l-dopa?
5. What can be the adverse side effects of l-dopa treatment?
6. What is postencephalitic parkinsonism?
7. About what percentage of individuals with idiopathic Parkinsons disease eventually develop dementia?
8. What is the most common phonation deficit in individuals with hypokinetic dysarthria?
9. Describe two rate control treatment tasks for individuals with increased rate of speech?
10. Describe two treatment tasks for reducing the harsh or breathy vocal quality that is so common in hypokinetic dysarthria.

CHAPTER

9

Hyperkinetic Dysarthria

DEFINITIONS OF HYPERKINETIC DYSARTHRIA

Hyperkinetic dysarthria is difficult to define, because it can be caused by so many disorders. Unlike hypokinetic dysarthria, which is so often caused by parkinsonism, hyperkinetic dysarthria can be caused by a long list of disorders. All of these disorders do have a few factors in common, however. Most of them seem to be caused by dysfunction in the basal ganglia, and they all produce involuntary movements that interfere with normal speech production.

> [A] dysarthria in which involuntary movements are present . . . muscle tone is abnormal, ranging from hypotonic to hypertonic, and, in some cases, fluctuating between the two. It includes various subclassifications, all of which are marked by disorders of loudness, rate, and inappropriate interruption of phonation. (Nicolosi et al., 1983, p. 80)

> Hyperkinetic dysarthria is characterized by variable articulatory imprecision, vocal harshness, and prosodic abnormalities. It is associated with damage to the extrapyramidal system, more specifically, lesions in the basal ganglia and their major pathways, which are important in the planning and programming of learned movements. (Zraick & LaPointe, 1997, p. 251)

In contrast to *hypokinetic*, which literally means too little movement, *hyperkinetic* means too much movement. Hyperkinetic movement disorders are characterized by excessive involuntary movements of various body parts. Chorea, myoclonus, tics, dystonia, and essential tremor are all examples of hyperkinetic movement disorders. The involuntary movements associated with these disorders frequently interfere with an affected individual's voluntary movements. When these involuntary movements interfere with speech production, the result is hyperkinetic dysarthria. Hyperkinetic dysarthria is unique among the other dysarthrias in that a clinician can often make an accurate diagnosis by just observing the individual's uncontrolled movements (Duffy, 1995).

Hyperkinetic movement disorders include many different involuntary motions, ranging from subtle movements of the lips, hands, or vocal folds to very large movements that involve many parts of the body. Every hyperkinetic disorder has its own characteristic movement pattern, with each resulting in distinctive patterns of speech errors. For example, the rapid and jerky muscle contractions of myoclonus cause different speech errors than the slow sustained muscle contractions of dystonia. Consequently, hyperkinetic dysarthria is actually a group of various motor speech disorders, with each being associated with one of the hyperkinetic movement disorders. For example, when describing the dysarthria of an individual with myoclonus or dystonia, it is more accurate to speak of the hyperkinetic dysarthria of myoclonus or the hyperkinetic dysarthria of dystonia than it is to use only the general term hyperkinetic dysarthria.

NEUROLOGICAL BASIS
OF HYPERKINETIC DYSARTHRIA

Many of the disorders that cause hyperkinetic dysarthria are associated with damage to the basal ganglia. As mentioned in previous chapters, the basal ganglia are a group of subcortical, gray matter structures that help control movements (Figure 9–1). The separate structures that make up the basal ganglia are the caudate nucleus, putamen, and the globus pallidus. The caudate nucleus and the putamen are together known as the striatum, because they share many of the same types of cells and many of the same functions. All the structures of the basal ganglia have a complex array of interconnections among themselves and with many other parts of the brain. One of these interconnections is a looping neural pathway that starts in the cerebral cortex, travels

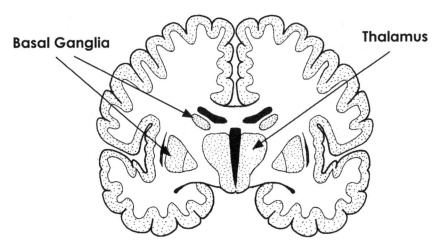

Basal Ganglia   **Thalamus**

Figure 9–1. Many hyperkinetic movement disorders are associated with damage to the basal ganglia. (Adapted from *Neuroscience of Communications* [p. 176], by D. Webster, 1999. San Diego: Singular Publishing Group, Inc. Copyright 1999 by Singular Publishing Group, Inc. Adapted with permission.)

down to the basal ganglia, and then goes back up to the cortical motor areas of the cerebrum. This pathway is called the basal ganglia control circuit (Figure 9–2).

The exact function of the basal ganglia and this control circuit are not fully understood, but these structures do play an important role in "smoothing out" the rough and exaggerated movements that are initially planned in the cerebral cortex. As discussed in Chapter 3, it is thought that the motor impulses of a planned movement are sent from the cortex to the basal ganglia, where the movements are processed and refined. Once these planned movements have been processed by

The Basal Ganglia Control Circuit

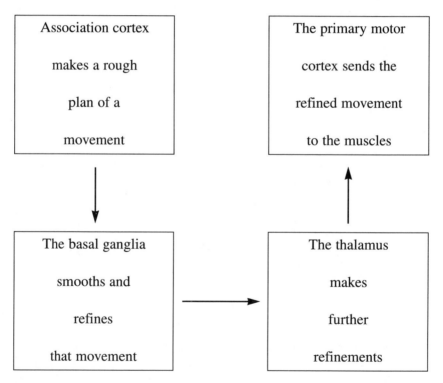

Figure 9–2. A schematic diagram of the basal ganglia control circuit.

the basal ganglia, they are sent back to the motor centers of the cortex (via the thalamus). From the motor centers of the cortex, these motor impulses are sent out to the upper motor neurons and then to the lower motor neurons. At the neuromuscular junction, the lower motor neurons transmit the neural impulses of the movement to the muscles, which then contract and perform the movement.

What Causes Hyperkinetic Movement?

Even though most hyperkinetic movement disorders seem to be associated with damage to the basal ganglia, neuroscientists have difficulty explaining exactly why the involuntary movements occur. For the most part, this is because the researchers are not yet sure how the basal ganglia functions. As with all complex mechanisms, it is much harder to determine why something is not working properly when its normal function is not well understood.

Although much remains to be learned about hyperkinetic movements, several important observations have been made about the workings of the basal ganglia. One is that different disorders associated with the basal ganglia can have nearly opposite effects on movements. Parkinsonism and Huntington's disease are two good examples of this. Both disorders are centered in the basal ganglia, yet the motor symptoms of each are very different. Parkinsonism is a hypokinetic disorder and is characterized by rigid and restricted movements. In contrast, Huntington's disease is a hyperkinetic disorder, characterized by rapid, dancelike involuntary movements. How is it that these two disorders of the basal ganglia have such different effects on movement?

Currently, it is the parkinsonism portion of this question that is best understood. As discussed in the previous chapter, parkinsonism is caused by the degeneration of dopamine-producing neurons near the striatum. The loss of these neurons reduces the amount of dopamine in the striatum. Decreased amounts of dopamine in these areas of the basal ganglia ultimately cause a diminution of movements. As a result, individuals with parkinsonism demonstrate the rigidity, akinesia, and other symptoms of the disorder.

Although this dopamine-deficiency explanation of the symptoms of parkinsonism is widely accepted, the causes of the symptoms of hyperkinetic movement disorders are less well understood. One theory suggests that the excessive involuntary movements in some of these disorders is caused by an imbalance of either dopamine or acetylcholine in the basal ganglia—an imbalance that is the inverse of that which causes parkinsonism. For example, any condition that causes too much dopamine to be released into the basal ganglia has an excitatory effect on movement. Similarly, any condition that causes too little acetylcholine in the basal ganglia also has an excitatory effect on movement. In either condition, hyperkinetic movements can be the result. This theory is supported by the experience of individuals with parkinsonism given too much l-dopa (i.e., too much dopamine) developing hyperkinetic movements (Wiederholt, 1995).

However, research indicates that the true cause of hyperkinetic movements is probably much more complicated than a simple imbalance of one or two neurotransmitters. The complexity of the basal ganglia can be appreciated from the fact that there are more than 100 different neuroactive chemicals in the striatum, alone (Brodal, 1992). The functions and interactions of these many chemicals are largely unknown, but they undoubtedly play varied roles in the proper functioning of the basal ganglia. Research suggests that the involuntary movements of hyperkinetic disorders are caused in part by disruptions in many of these neurochemicals, although the process is far from being fully understood. Until the intricate functions of the basal ganglia are better comprehended, the exact reasons for the involuntary movements of hyperkinetic disorders will remain unclear.

ETIOLOGIES OF HYPERKINETIC DYSARTHRIA

Several hyperkinetic movement disorders can lead to hyperkinetic dysarthria. The disorders examined in this chapter are chorea, myoclonus, tics, essential tremor, and dystonia. As mentioned, most of these hyperkinetic movement disorders are associated with damage to the basal ganglia, the basal ganglia control circuit, or both. Degenerative diseases, traumatic head injury, stroke, infections, and other etiologies can cause this damage. However, some of the hyperkinetic disorders, such as essential tremor, seem to have no observable neurological pathology associated with them.

The involuntary movements linked to hyperkinetic disorders can vary, both in severity and in type of movement. In mild cases, the movements may be small tremors of one muscle. In severe cases, the movements may be so pronounced and affect so much of the body that such activities as walking, eating, and talking are practically impossible. Naturally, there can be definite differences between the dysarthria associated with mild tremor and the dysarthria associated with extreme involuntary movements of large muscle groups.

The overall impression of hyperkinetic dysarthria is that involuntary movements are interfering with an affected individual's efforts to produce speech (Duffy, 1995). A further impression is that speech production might be normal if the involuntary movements would somehow cease. The specific characteristics of the hyperkinetic dysarthria associated with each of the hyperkinetic movement disorders is discussed in the following sections of this chapter. Most of the information will concentrate on the hyperkinetic dysarthria associated with chorea and dystonia, because the speech disorders of these two conditions are the most fully documented.

Chorea

Chorea is a movement disorder distinguished by random involuntary movements of the limbs, trunk, head, and neck. Choreic motions are often described as dancelike, because they appear to be smooth and coordinated. In fact, the term comes from *choreia*, the Greek word for dance, which incidentally also is the root of the word choreography. Although choreic movements may seem to be coordinated, they are actually unpredictable and purposeless. They are sometimes even jerky or abrupt. Other descriptions of chorea have characterized the movements as writhing, highly complex, fleeting, and irregular. In mild cases of chorea, the motions might not be immediately obvious to an observer; they may give the impression that the affected individual is only restless or jittery. When the movements are infrequent, the affected individual may try to hide them by turning them into purposeful gestures, such as scratching the chin or stretching an arm. In severe cases, the motions are constant, stopping only when the individual is asleep. When they are severe, the choreic motions will interfere with nearly all attempts at voluntary movement. As a result, problems with walking, swallowing, speech, and other discrete movements are common in individuals with advanced chorea.

Sydenham's Chorea

Chorea is the shared symptom of several neurologic disorders. One of these disorders is Sydenham's chorea, a rare disorder that affects children between 5 and 15 years of age. The familiar name for this condition is St. Vitus dance. Its occurrence is closely associated with children who have had rheumatic fever. The cause of Sydenham's chorea is unknown. It may be caused in part by hypersensitive dopamine receptors in the basal ganglia or by too much dopamine in these same areas of the brain. About 40% of the children with this disorder have the hyperkinetic dysarthria of chorea. Fortunately, Sydenham's chorea usually clears in 3 to 4 months without treatment.

Huntington's Disease

Huntington's disease is a progressive disorder that is caused by the gradual degeneration of neurons in the basal ganglia and cerebral cortex. The loss of neurons is especially evident in the caudate nucleus and putamen (the striatum) in the basal ganglia. Huntington disease is an inherited (autosomal dominant) disorder, with half the children of an affected individual developing the condition. Its prevalence is about 6 per 100,000. Although the first signs of the disease can appear in childhood or adolescence, the typical age of onset is middle age. The average course of the disease is about 15 years, but some individuals survive for 25 or 30 years after the symptoms first appear.

The clinical features and progression of Huntington's disease are very unfortunate. The earliest signs are subtle intellectual deficits that may be only evident in neuropsychological testing. For example, performance scores on the *Wechsler Adult Intelligence Scale* may decline in affected individuals for months or years before other symptoms of the disease are apparent. Inevitably, a significant dementia will develop, in which patients show personality changes, impaired problem solving abilities, and word-finding difficulties. Individuals with Huntington disease eventually become inattentive, vague, withdrawn, and depressed. Angry outbursts and suicidal thoughts are not unusual. Along with this cognitive decline, a generalized chorea develops as the loss of basal ganglia neurons progresses. The choreic movements interfere with voluntary actions, resulting in a lurching walk, poorly coordinated fine motor movements, dysphagia, and hyperkinetic dysarthria. In the final stages of the disease, many individuals with Huntington's disease are bedridden, mute, and akinetic (Lechtenberg, 1982).

The cause of the neuron degeneration in Huntington's disease is unclear. Several theories have been proposed, including the hypothesis that the affected person's brain produces a toxin that kills the neurons (Brodal, 1992). It is known, however, that the loss of these neurons accompanies significant decreases in certain neurotransmitter receptors in the basal ganglia and reductions in important enzymes and other neuroactive chemicals in the brain. These complex neurological changes are thought to be responsible for many of the symptoms of this disease, although researchers are uncertain precisely how the loss of neurons in the striatum causes choreic movements.

Stroke

Although it is rare, strokes have been known to cause chorea (Warlow, 1991). Usually, these are strokes affecting the basal ganglia or nearby subcortical structures such as the thalamus. The resulting chorea is commonly called hemichorea because the involuntary movements occur only on the side of the body that is opposite to the site of the lesion, assuming that the stroke damage is restricted to only one side of the brain.

Sometimes, stroke damage to the subthalamic nucleus, a collection of subcortical motor neurons near the substantia nigra, can cause a condition known as **hemiballism**. This disorder is characterized by wild and violent involuntary movements of the limbs that are contralateral to the lesion. Although this disorder is a distinct diagnostic category from chorea, hemiballistic movements are described occasionally as being extreme versions of choreic movements. Self-injury and exhaustion are very possible in cases of hemiballism. In most instances, the movements can be treated successfully with medications, and they usually remit spontaneously after a period of days, weeks, or months.

Tardive Dyskinesia

Tardive dyskinesia is a movement disorder that can cause choreic movements of the face, mouth, and neck. In some instances the limbs also are affected. Tardive dyskinesia is caused by taking certain antipsychotic (neuroleptic) drugs over a period of months or years. The term tardive dyskinesia is an apt description of this disorder, because the choreic movements appear after long-term use of these drugs. (Tardive means being late in appearing, as in being tardy; dyskinesia means a disorder of voluntary movement.) Women are more likely to develop this condition than men are, and elderly individuals are more susceptible than the young. Unfortunately, stopping the medications will not reverse the condition in most cases. In fact, tardive dyskinesia will sometimes appear only after the medications are withdrawn, a condition known as withdrawal-emergent dyskinesia.

The movements of the face and mouth in tardive dyskinesia include lip smacking, tongue protrusions, chewing motions, and grimacing (Warlow, 1991). Such movements can cause hyperkinetic dysarthria by interfering with normal voluntary attempts at speech production. It is not exactly clear why these drugs cause hyperkinetic movements. It is thought that they may make certain neurotransmitter receptors in neurons of the basal ganglia supersensitive to dopamine.

As a consequence, the basal ganglia will react as if it were receiving too much dopamine even if only normal amounts are present. The result is an excessively excitatory effect on movement.

Other Causes of Chorea

Several other conditions can cause choreic movements. These include cerebral anoxia and carbon monoxide poisoning. Both injuries can selectively damage the basal ganglia and other related subcortical structures, although chorea is not a typical symptom of either condition. Pregnancy and the use of oral contraceptives also can cause chorea, but the incidence is very low.

Speech Characteristics of Hyperkinetic Dysarthria of Chorea

Chorea can have a significant effect on speech production. Of course, the severity of the chorea influences how severely speech is affected. Individuals with mild chorea typically will have fewer speech errors than someone who is more significantly impaired. In fact, individuals with very mild cases of chorea may have minimal problems with their speech. In the more moderately and severely affected individuals, however, a wide variety of speech errors will be evident. The variety of errors is primarily based on two factors. First, the movements of chorea may affect many different muscle groups, including the muscles of the face, neck, head, and torso. The voluntary movements of all of these muscles are susceptible to interference from the involuntary movements of chorea. As a consequence, *all* the components of speech production (articulation, phonation, respiration, resonance, and prosody) may be more or less equally affected by hyperkinetic movements. This is in contrast to many of the other dysarthrias, in which at least one of the components of speech production is usually less affected than the others are. For example, in spastic dysarthria respiration is usually far less impaired than phonation and articulation.

Second, the movements of chorea are unpredictable. At a given moment, the choreic movements may affect any number of muscle groups. For instance, during speech, the muscles of the lips and tongue may be affected for one instant, and at the next instant, the muscles of respiration will cause a sudden inhalation of air during phonation. A moment later, yet another muscle group may be affected. It also is possible that all the muscles of speech production will be affected simultaneously by the involuntary movements. On the other hand, there may be short periods in which the interference from the choreic movements is minimal. At those moments, speech production may be acceptably good, if only briefly.

The following paragraphs examine the effects of chorea on each component of speech production, based mostly on Darley et al.'s (1969a, 1969b) analysis of the speech errors of 30 subjects with chorea. The complete ranking of the speech errors is presented in Table 9–1. Note that a few of the errors appear to be contradictory, such as monoloudness and excess loudness variations. In general, such errors reflect the variability and unpredictable nature of choreic movements, which can cause, for instance, both monoloudness and excessive loudness in the same individual at different times.

Table 9–1. The Most Common Speech Production Errors in 30 Individuals With Hyperkinetic Dysarthria of Chorea

Rank	Speech Production Errors
1	Imprecise consonants
2	Prolonged intervals
3	Variable pitch
4	Monopitch
5	Harsh voice quality
6	Inappropriate silences
7	Distorted vowels
8	Excess loudness variation
9	Prolonged phonemes
10	Monoloudness
11	Short phrases
12.5	Irregular articulatory breakdown
12.5	Excess and equal stress
14.5	Hypernasality
14.5	Reduced stress
16	Strained-strangled quality

Source: From "Clusters of Diagnostic Patterns of Dysarthria," by F. L. Darley, A. E. Aronson, and J. R. Brown, 1969, *Journal of Speech and Hearing Research, 12*, p. 260. Copyright 1969 by American Speech-Language-Hearing Association. Reprinted with permission.

Prosody

Darley et al. found that chorea affects prosody more than any other component of speech production. The two prosodic errors that were most evident in their subjects were **prolonged intervals** between syllables and words and **variable rate** of speech. Duffy (1995) suggested that these errors are caused by the unpredictable timing of the choreic movements and by an individual's attempts to compensate for the movements. For example, an individual may wait for the completion of an interfering choreic motion before continuing with an utterance. This would cause a prolonged time interval between syllables or words. On the other hand, a speaker could hurry through an utterance before the next choreic movement occurs and thus have a variable rate of speech. Some of the other noted prosodic errors are **monopitch**, **inappropriate silences**, and **monoloudness**.

Articulation

Imprecise consonants, distorted vowels, and **prolonged phonemes** were common articulation errors in Darley et al.'s (1969a, 1969b) subjects with chorea. The first two of these articulation errors are the result of involuntary choreic movements being imposed on the voluntary movements of normal articulation. For example, involuntary contractions of the pharyngeal muscles may change the shape of the vocal tract during speech and thereby cause any vowel spoken at that moment to be distorted. The third articulation error, prolongation of phonemes, can be caused by choreic movements that involuntarily force the holding of an articulatory position longer than is normally required.

Phonation

Choreic movements also can affect phonation. Darley et al. (1969a, 1969b) found **harsh vocal quality, excess loudness variations,** and **strained-strangled vocal quality** in many of their subjects. These errors of phonation are caused by intermittent, involuntary hyperadduction of the vocal folds during speech. On the other hand, involuntary vocal fold abduction during phonation can cause brief instances of **breathy vocal quality**. In fact, some individuals with chorea may demonstrate a harsh or strained-strangled vocal quality in one utterance and then have a breathy vocal quality in a portion of the next one. As mentioned, such variability reflects the unpredictable nature of choreic movements. At one moment, the vocal folds might be adducted too tightly; shortly afterwards, they may be unable to adduct fully. Choreic movements also may cause instances of **voice stoppage** in which phonation ceases intermittently during speech.

Respiration

Darley et al. (1969a, 1969b) reported that six of their subjects with chorea had rapid, **unexpected inhalations** and **exhalations** of air. These sudden respiratory actions are caused by involuntary movements of the chest or diaphragm. In severe cases of chorea, these respiratory actions can occur at any moment, either while sitting quietly or in the middle of an utterance. During speech, they can cause distracting extraneous phonations, halting utterances, and short phrases. By causing a sudden increase in subglottic air pressure, involuntary exhalations during phonation can contribute to the excess loudness variations noted in the previous paragraph.

Resonance

Hypernasality was noted in 13 of Darley et al.'s subjects. This problem of resonance is caused by involuntary movements that alter the normal timing of velar elevation. Duffy (1995) indicated that hypernasality in chorea is usually intermittent, which reflects the unpredictable nature of the movements. Brief moments of hyponasality also are possible, caused by involuntary velar movements that close the velopharyngeal port during the production of nasal phonemes.

Summary of Distinctive Speech Errors in Chorea

There are many speech errors that can occur in the hyperkinetic dysarthria of chorea. There are so many, in fact, that beginning clinicians can be overwhelmed and confused by their number. To simplify this situation, the following list summarizes speech errors that are generally most evident in individuals with chorea (Duffy, 1995):

- Prolonged intervals between syllables and words
- Variable rate of speech
- Inappropriate silences
- Excess loudness variations
- Prolonged phonemes
- Rapid, brief inhalations or exhalations of air

- Voice stoppages
- Intermittent breathy voice quality

Myoclonus

Myoclonus is a hyperkinetic movement disorder distinguished by involuntary and brief contractions of part of a muscle, a whole muscle, or a group of muscles in the same area of the body. *Myo* means muscle; *clonus* means alternating contraction and relaxation (*Clonus* is from the Greek word for turmoil). The muscle contractions of myoclonus may occur singly, in a repeating irregular pattern, or rhythmically. Furthermore, these contractions cannot be suppressed consciously. Myoclonus can appear as part of many medical conditions. It can be found in cases of kidney failure, epilepsy, cerebral anoxia, strokes, traumatic head injury, and some progressive neurological diseases such as Alzheimer disease or Creutzfeldt-Jakob disease. It also can appear for unknown reasons. This disorder is not always disabling. In fact, nearly everyone has experienced benign hypnagogic myoclonus, which is the whole-body jerk that sometimes happens immediately before falling to sleep.

A focal myoclonus occurs when specific muscles or body parts are affected by the contractions. **Hemifacial spasm** is a good example of a focal myoclonus. In this condition, there are involuntary contractions of the muscles around the eye. These contractions may eventually spread to other muscles until nearly all of the muscles on the same side of the face are affected. It is a common disorder and is painless, but the social consequences of embarrassment can be significant.

Another example of a focal myoclonus is **palatopharyngolaryngeal myoclonus**, sometimes less accurately known as just palatal myoclonus. Unlike hemifacial spasm, this condition is rare. As its name implies, palatopharyngolaryngeal myoclonus is marked by muscular contractions of the soft palate, the pharynx, and the larynx. The contractions are fairly rhythmic and occur about 1–3 times a second, even while sleeping (Warlow, 1991). Brainstem strokes are the most likely cause of this condition, but other etiologies include cerebellar lesions, encephalitis, and tumors. In many cases, the cause is unknown.

Soft palate contractions are the most frequently noted movement in palatopharyngolaryngeal myoclonus. They consist of brief and rapid elevating contractions that often can be easily observed. The associated contractions of the pharynx can be seen as rhythmic movements of the pharyngeal walls. Interestingly, these pharyngeal contrac tions can repeatedly open and close the eustachian tube, which causes an audible (and to the affected individual, a very annoying) clicking sound. The laryngeal contractions of this disorder can sometimes be visible as a twitching of the neck muscles. The effects of palatopharyngolaryngeal myoclonus on speech production are less obvious than might be surmised by the many involuntary movements associated with it. Speech is affected in only the most severe cases of this disorder, because the contractions are typically so quick and of such a low intensity (Duffy, 1995). Darley et al. (1975) reported that when speech is involved, there might be intermittent hypernasality, imprecise consonants, and short interruptions of phonation.

Tic Disorders

A tic is a rapid movement that can be controlled voluntarily for a certain period, but nevertheless is performed frequently because of a compulsive desire to do so. Affected individuals report that they can suppress a tic for varying lengths of time, but the urge to perform the movement builds irresistibly until they are compelled to do it. There are both motor tics and vocal tics. The most common motor tics involve the face, such as repetitive eye blinks, brief facial twitches, or grimaces. However, motor tics also can be more obvious and complex, revealing themselves as hand gestures, squatting, kicking, hopping, or shoulder shrugging. Vocal tics may take the form of throat clearing, grunts, or barking noises. Extreme examples of vocal tics include shouting and the compulsive utterance of obscene words (coprolalia). Stress often increases the frequency of tic behaviors.

The etiology of some tics can be traced to mild brain damage or toxic reactions to medications, but there is no identifiable CNS disorder in most cases (Lechtenberg, 1982). These idiopathic tics occur in about 10% to 12% of all children, usually in the form of excessive eyeblinks or other brief facial movements. In affected children, the tics may occur for less than a month or up to about a year, after which most disappear. Sometimes, however, a tic will persist. In fact, it may be joined by other tic behaviors over time.

Multiple motor and vocal tics are one of the four clinical features of **Gilles de la Tourette syndrome**, which is a rare tic disorder that was first identified in 1825. The other three clinical features of Tourette syndrome are (a) the development of symptoms before the age of 14, (b) the slow appearance and disappearance of symptoms, and (c) tic behaviors that change and evolve over time (Lechtenberg, 1982).

Although no specific organic etiology has been identified in Tourette syndrome, minor neurological abnormalities have been noted in some affected people (Wiederholt, 1995). One theory suggests that this disorder is caused by supersensitive dopamine receptors in the striatum. There appears to a family link in about 35% of cases. Almost all children who are diagnosed with this disorder show definite symptoms by age 10. The prevalence of Tourette syndrome is about 3 per 100,000 of the general population, with boys being affected far more frequently than girls.

The motor and vocal tics found in Tourette syndrome can include all of those mentioned previously. In addition, such vocal tics as palilalia (the compulsive repetition of one's own speech) and echolalia (the compulsive repetition of someone else's speech) can appear in this disorder. Tourette syndrome is often accompanied by obsessive-compulsive behaviors.

Essential (or Organic) Tremor

Essential tremor is a benign hyperkinetic movement disorder that causes tremulous movements in affected body parts. The terms essential and organic are often used synonymously in labeling this disorder. In this context, both terms mean that a disorder has no apparent external cause (i.e., it is idiopathic). Essential tremor is the most common hyperkinetic movement disorder seen by neurologists, occurring in about 300 per 100,000 of the population. It usually first appears when individuals are in their 40s or 50s, but it has been first noted at much younger and older ages. About 50% of the individuals with essential tremor have family members who also show signs of this disorder, hence the use of the term *familial tremor* to sometimes describe this tremor.

Essential tremor most often affects the hands, arms, or head. It is an action tremor, which means that it is most evident when an individual is performing a movement, such as lifting a glass to the mouth or writing. When the affected body part is at rest, the tremor disappears or is greatly reduced. Stress and fatigue will increase the tremor. Although most cases of essential tremor have a gradual onset, sudden onset of this condition has been noted. Once the tremor does appear, any progression of severity typically occurs at a slow pace. As its name implies, no specific site of lesion has been identified for this disorder, but it has been occasionally associated with hemifacial spasm and focal dystonia (discussed shortly). Although essential tremor is occasionally confused with parkinsonian tremor, Wiederholt (1995) indicated three characteristics that help distinguish between them:

- Essential tremor is faster than that of parkinsonism tremor.
- Essential tremor is an action tremor that disappears at rest; parkinsonian tremor is a resting tremor that decreases during movement.
- Individuals with essential tremor do not have other neurologic symptoms such a bradykinesia, akinesia, dementia, and so forth.

Essential *voice* tremor occurs in about 20% of individuals with essential tremor (Jankovic, 1990, as cited in Duffy, 1995). It is characterized by phonation that has a tremulous, quavering vocal quality. This tremulous quality is caused by rhythmic, involuntary contractions of the vocal folds, along with vertical laryngeal movements (Aronson, 1990). These contractions occur at a rate of about 6 per second. There is a wide severity range in essential voice tremor. In mild cases, the tremor will be "hidden" by the vigorous vocal tract movements of conversational speech and be evident only during a prolonged vowel. In fact, Duffy (1995) indicated that some individuals with mild essential voice tremor are not aware that they have the condition. In the more severe cases, tremor of the lips, tongue, or neck may accompany the rhythmic contractions of the larynx. All attempts at phonation will have a clearly evident tremulous quality. If severe enough, these vocal tract tremors may slow the rate of speech in affected individuals.

Dystonia

Dystonia is a hyperkinetic movement disorder of muscle tone. *Dys* means disordered or abnormal; *tonia* is muscle tone. Dystonia causes involuntary, prolonged muscle contractions that interfere with normal movement or posture. Dystonic movements typically have a slower, more sustained quality than those seen in chorea. Because the effect of dystonia is not necessarily constant, dystonic muscular contractions may appear and disappear during an ongoing movement. These gradual changes in muscle tone are described often as the "waxing and waning" characteristic of dystonia. In severe cases, however, the contractions can be constant, often resulting in painful, fixed contractions of the affected body part. For example, in a severe case of tongue dystonia, the tongue may protrude fully in a very strong and steady muscular contraction, making all attempts at speech uncomfortable and practically impossible.

Dystonia can appear in many muscles of the body. It may affect only one muscle, a single group of muscles, or multiple groups of muscles. Dystonia is categorized according to the number of affected body parts (Warlow, 1991):

- **Focal dystonia**—when the dystonic movement or posture is present in only one part of the body, such as the tongue, arm, or hand.
- **Segmental dystonia**—when the dystonic movement or posture includes two or more parts of the body, such as in Meige syndrome (to be discussed) in which the dystonic movements affect the neck, larynx, soft palate, jaw, and face.
- **Generalized dystonia**—when the dystonic movement or posture affect all four limbs and the torso or neck.
- **Hemidystonia**—when the dystonic movement or posture affect two or more body parts on the same side of the body.

Sometimes dystonic muscular contractions can be alleviated temporarily by **sensory tricks**. Sensory tricks are simple movements or actions that an affected individual can perform to stop the involuntary contractions—at least for a short period. Sensory tricks are very idiosyncratic. A trick that works for one person may have no effect for someone else. A frequently reported sensory trick is a gentle touch to the affected body part. For example, in a case of mandibular dystonia, the sensory trick of lightly touching the jaw may temporarily stop the involuntary muscular contractions. Usually, individuals with dystonia find effective sensory tricks either by accident or experimentation. In one case study, an individual with dystonia of the tongue found that when he put a breath mint between his cheek and gum, his dystonic tongue movements would stop until the mint dissolved. While the mint was in his mouth, his speech articulation was normal. Unfortunately, the dystonic movements of some individuals do not respond to sensory tricks. Even when they do work, sensory tricks tend to lose their effectiveness after long-term use. The reason why they work at all is a mystery.

Etiologies of Dystonia

Dystonia can result from numerous conditions including focal CVAs of the basal ganglia, traumatic head injury, carbon monoxide poisoning, cerebral anoxia, and tumors. In these conditions, dystonia can be just one of several symptoms (i.e., a secondary symptom). There also are disorders where dystonia is the primary symptom. These disorders are known as **primary dystonias**.

Spasmodic Torticollis

Spasmodic torticollis is a good example of a primary dystonia. This disorder is characterized by intermittent dystonic contractions of the neck muscles, which result in an involuntary turning of the head. The head also usually tilts upward as a result of the contractions. In some cases, spasmodic torticollis eventually develops into a generalized dystonia. The contractions in this disorder are intermittent, meaning that for varying amounts of time there will be no evidence of dystonia. However, stress and anxiety tend to increase the frequency of the contractions. In some individuals, the sensory trick of gently touching the turned-away side of the face can stop the neck muscle contractions and allow normal movement for a time. The cause of spasmodic torticollis is unknown, but basal ganglia neuron degeneration has been noted in some individuals with the disorder. The speech of affected individuals has been shown to be slow in rate, mildly reduced in intelligibility, and lower in pitch for many females (Duffy, 1995).

Drug-Induced Dystonia

In addition to causing the choreic movements of tardive dyskinesia, the long-term use of certain antipsychotic drugs also can result in a primary dystonia known as **chronic drug-induced dystonia**. As in tardive dyskinesia, withdrawal of the drug may not stop the dystonia. In fact in some cases, the dystonia may appear only after the drug has been withdrawn. Most of the dystonic contractions in this disorder appear near the mouth and face, resulting in grimacing, sustained tongue protrusions, and so forth. Occasionally, the dystonic movements will generalize to other body parts. Drug-induced dystonia also is known as **tardive dystonia**.

Meige's Syndrome

Meige's syndrome is a rare idiopathic disease. One of the most prominent symptoms is repetitive eyeblinking and abnormal facial movements that are often dystonic in nature. The first signs of this disorder appear in early middle age and get progressively worse. The eye blinks can become so frequent that functional vision is impossible. The involuntary facial movements of this disease can affect the jaw, tongue, mouth, and neck. When the dystonic facial movements are sufficiently strong, they often cause hyperkinetic dysarthria.

Spasmodic Dysphonia

Although it is not always classified as a primary dystonia, spasmodic dysphonia has many of the features of a focal dystonia. This disorder is characterized by involuntary vocal fold movements during phonation. Unlike a typical dystonia, the muscular contractions of spasmodic dysphonia do not usually have a gradual waxing and waning quality. Rather, the involuntary movements are frequently described as being vigorous and active. In a majority of individuals, the spasmodic movements affect the adductor muscles in the larynx—causing what is known as adductor spasmodic dysphonia. In this condition, the vocal folds are involuntarily closed tightly during phonation. This involuntary adduction of the vocal folds can be either constant or intermittent. When it is constant, an affected person's phonations typically have a continuously strained and effortful quality. When the adduction is intermittent, phonations have a jerky and tight quality. In mild cases, phonations may have only a modestly "shaky" quality. In the less common abductor form of spasmodic dysphonia, the vocal folds are involuntarily abducted during phonation—resulting in moments of breathiness or aphonia.

An interesting feature of this disorder is that nonlinguistic vocalizations such as laughing or crying are free of the involuntary laryngeal contractions. Many spontaneous, emotionally charged vocalizations also are clear of the dysphonia. This unusual feature of spasmodic dysphonia led many early investigators to assume that its etiology was psychogenic. Currently, it is believed that most cases of this disorder probably have a neurogenic origin, although the pathological process causing the involuntary vocal fold movements is unclear. Its closeness to a focal dystonia suggests that the cause may be related to a basal ganglia disorder.

Speech Characteristics of Hyperkinetic Dysarthria of Dystonia

Darley et al. (1969a, 1969b) examined the speech errors of 30 subjects with dystonia (see Table 9–2). Numerous errors were noted, many of which also were present in their subjects with chorea. The apparent similarity of speech errors in dystonia and chorea can be confusing to

Table 9–2. The Most Common Speech Production Errors in 30 Individuals With the Hyperkinetic Dysarthria of Dystonia

Rank	Speech Production Errors
1	Imprecise consonants
2	Distorted vowels
3	Harsh voice quality
4	Irregular articulatory breakdown
5.5	Strained-strangled quality
5.5	Monopitch
7	Monoloudness
8.5	Inappropriate silences
8.5	Short phrases
10	Prolonged intervals
11	Prolonged phonemes
12	Excess loudness variation
13	Reduced stress
14	Voice stoppages
15	Rate

Source: From "Clusters of Diagnostic Patterns of Dysarthria," by F. L. Darley, A. E. Aronson, and J. R. Brown, 1969, *Journal of Speech and Hearing Research, 12,* p. 259. Copyright 1969 by American Speech-Language-Hearing Association. Reprinted with permission.

many clinicians. However, a careful comparison of Tables 9–1 and 9–2 reveals several important distinctions between these two hyperkinetic disorders. First, Darley et al. found more errors of articulation in dystonia than in chorea. Three of the top four errors in dystonia were articulation errors; there was only one articulation error (imprecise consonants) in the top four for chorea. Second, the subjects with chorea tended to display more prosodic errors than those with dystonia. Three of the top four errors in chorea were errors of prosody; no prosodic errors were in the top four errors in the subjects with dystonia. In general, the speech errors in individuals with chorea tend to reflect errors of prosody, and those in individuals with dystonia tend to reflect errors of articulation. Although such distinctions may be somewhat helpful in diagnosing these two forms of hyperkinetic dysarthria, it should be remembered that there will always be numerous individuals with either disorder who do not precisely match these patterns of speech errors.

Articulation

As mentioned, Darley et al. found that articulation errors were the most prominent in their subjects with dystonia. **Imprecise consonants, distorted vowels, irregular articulatory breakdowns,** and **prolonged phonemes** were evident in their subjects' speech. These errors are the result of sustained dystonic contractions of the oral motor muscles that cause incorrect or imprecise positioning of the articulators during speech. The irregular articulatory breakdowns reflect the intermittent nature of many dystonic contractions. When they are present during speech, dystonic movements will interfere with accurate articulation; when they are absent, articulation will be improved considerably.

Prosody

Although typically less prominent than articulation errors, prosodic errors can occur frequently in dystonia. Darley et al.'s (1969a, 1969b) subjects demonstrated **monopitch, monoloudness, inappropriate silences,** and **short phrases**. They also tended to reduce stress on normally stressed words and syllables. Many of these prosodic errors may be the result of dystonic muscular contractions in the vocal tract that reduce the range and speed of the laryngeal movements needed to produce normal inflections of pitch and loudness.

Phonation

Darley et al. found a **harsh vocal quality** in 27 of their 30 subjects with dystonia. Many of them also had **strained-strangled quality** as well. These phonation problems are probably caused by increased muscle tone in the larynx, which results in a tighter, narrower glottal opening during speech. **Excessive loudness variation** also was noted in some of the subjects. As in chorea, excessive loudness variation is most likely the result of momentary hyperadduction of the vocal folds during speech. The cooccurrence of both monoloudness and excessive loudness variation in some individuals with dystonia is explained by the unpredictable waxing and waning quality of dystonic muscular contractions in the larynx. Respiration deficits also may be a factor in these loudness changes (see next paragraph).

Respiration

Respiratory problems are not common in dystonia. However, Duffy (1995) suggested that the excessive loudness variation might be due to the effects of dystonia on respiration. This increase in loudness may be caused directly by dystonic movements that involuntarily contract the respiratory muscles during phonation. It also may be caused indirectly by an affected individual attempting to compensate for abnormal respiratory movements. In either situation, the result could be excessive changes in loudness during speech.

Resonance

Hypernasality was present in 11 of Darley et al.'s (1969a, 1969b) 30 subjects with dystonia; however, it was not severe enough to be included in their ranking of speech errors. This low rating suggests that although hypernasality may be present in dystonia, it is most often quite mild.

KEY EVALUATION TASKS FOR HYPERKINETIC DYSARTHRIA

1. Vowel prolongation is useful in detecting the harsh or strained-strangled vocal quality that can be present in several of the hyperkinetic dysarthrias. It also may be helpful in evoking a vocal tremor, especially when the tremor is mild. In addition, vowel prolongation can be useful in determining pitch and loudness variations that may be caused by involuntary contractions of the oral, laryngeal, and respiratory muscles.
2. Duffy (1995) suggested that alternate motion rates can highlight the irregular articulatory breakdowns and speech rate variations that can occur in the hyperkinetic dysarthrias.
3. Conversational speech and reading materials may provide the most comprehensive picture of the speech in individuals with hyperkinetic dysarthria. These two tasks can evoke articulatory errors (e.g., imprecise consonants, vowel distortions, and prolonged phonemes), prosodic errors (e.g., silences, monopitch, monoloudness, short phrases), phonatory errors (e.g., harshness, excessive loudness variations) and respiratory errors (e.g., sudden inhalations or exhalations of air) that may occur in the speech of these individuals.
4. Careful observation of the associated involuntary movements is a critical part of evaluating hyperkinetic dysarthria. Each hyperkinetic disorder has its own general pattern of involuntary movements. The following outline highlights the primary distinctions of the hyperkinetic movement disorders mentioned in this chapter:

- **Chorea**—characterized by relatively quick, unpredictable, co-ordinated movements of the limbs, head, face, mouth, and neck; sometimes having a dancelike quality.
- **Myoclonus**—distinguished by brief contractions of a single muscle or body part. These contractions may occur singly, in a repeating irregular pattern, or rhythmically. Unlike tics, my-oclonic contractions cannot be consciously suppressed.
- **Tic disorders**—motor or vocal behaviors that can be controlled voluntarily until the compulsive desire to perform the behavior becomes overwhelming. Motor tics include eyeblinks, shoulder shrugs, and head jerks. Vocal tics include grunting, humming, and barking noises.
- **Essential tremor**—a benign action tremor that usually affects the hands, arms, or head. Essential tremor results in essential voice tremor when it affects the vocal folds.
- **Dystonia**—characterized by sustained, involuntary contractions of muscles in one or more body parts; these contractions often come and go in a waxing and waning pattern. Dystonic movements are usually slower and more prolonged than those seen in chorea.

TREATMENT OF HYPERKINETIC DYSARTHRIA

Most of the treatments for hyperkinetic dysarthria are medications that suppress the involuntary movements that cause the speech deficits. For example, choreic movements and tic behaviors can be reduced by haloperidol; myoclonic jerks can be treated with clonazepam or valproic acid. Unfortunately, no drug-based treatment for any of the hyperkinetic movement disorders has proven to be consistently effective for all patients with these disorders. In addition, most of these medications have significant adverse side effects. For instance, haloperidol can cause sleepiness and dystonic movements. It also can cause tardive dyskinesia if it is taken for prolonged periods.

Perhaps the most successful medication for a hyperkinetic disorder is Botox, which is used to treat spasmodic torticollis, spasmodic dysphonia, and several of the other dystonic movement disorders. This substance is a weakened form of the botulism toxin. By interfering with the transmission of acetylcholine across the neuromuscular junction, an injection of Botox into muscle tissue can greatly reduce dystonic contractions in affected muscles. Botox injections are usually effective for several months. Although they need to be repeated on a regular basis, Botox injections can provide significant relief for patients experiencing these dystonic movement disorders.

The following paragraphs discuss the behavior-based treatments for hyperkinetic dysarthria. These types of treatments for hyperkinetic dysarthria are worth a trial therapy period, if the patient is not too severely affected.

- **Sensory tricks**—Duffy (1995) recommended that clinicians encourage patients with dystonia to find and use sensory tricks that can suppress their involuntary movements. Given that some of these sensory tricks can be quite subtle and need not draw undue attention, this can be a relatively easy treatment option. The drawback, however, is that sensory tricks seldom have long-term effectiveness, nor do they work for every patient. Nevertheless, patients with dystonia should be told about sensory tricks if they have not discovered them for themselves.
- **Relaxation therapy and related treatments**—Several studies have examined the effectiveness of relaxation therapy, supportive psychotherapy, and mental imagery as treatments for the tic behaviors in Tourette syndrome (Bergin, Waranch, Brown, Carson, & Singer, 1998; Peterson & Cohen, 1998). The results of these studies have been inconclusive. For instance, the relaxation technique used by Bergin et al. taught the subjects to assume a relaxed bodily posture that included lightly closed eyelids, a relaxed neck and limbs, and no eye movements. The findings of this study, however, showed no long-term reduction in tic behavior. Moreover, the early reports of successful psychotherapy for tics (Mahler, Luke, & Daltroff, 1945) have not be replicated in later clinical investigations.

  However, several studies have demonstrated some reductions in tic behaviors through the use of behavioral techniques. Kohen and Botts (1987) used mental imagery to teach their four subjects to imagine pleasant scenes to create a feeling of being able to control their own experiences. The authors reported reduced tics in the subjects. Azrin and Peterson (1990) demonstrated a 30% to 50% decrease in tics through the use of a habit reversal procedure. The habit reversal procedure taught the subjects to use competing voluntary behaviors to prevent or interrupt the tics. For example, a subject with rapid eyeblink tics was taught to voluntarily blink slowly before the tics occurred. Although these two studies reported positive results, further research is needed into such treatments to replicate the findings.

- **Bite blocks**—A well-known treatment for focal dystonic jaw movements is the use of a bite block to stabilize the jaw during speech. A bite block is a small cube of plastic that the patient bites down upon during speech. The voluntary contractions of the jaw muscles that hold the block in place seem to suppress dystonic jaw movements in many patients. As a consequence, more stable articulatory contacts can be made while speaking because the jaw is stable. A bite block does not necessarily need to be visible, because it can be held between the molars in the back of the mouth.

- **Easy onset of phonation**—There is some anecdotal evidence that easy onset procedures can lessen involuntary movements affecting the larynx during speech but only in mild cases. The overall goal of the treatment is to have the patient make softer glottal closures while phonating. The first step asks the patient to exhale while producing a smooth, quiet sigh. Once these soft sighs are produced consistently, the patient is asked to gently initiate a prolonged phonation of an open vowel such as /a/. These prolonged phonations are then shaped into words that begin with vowels or breathy consonant such as /w/. The ultimate goal is to build toward easy phonations of sentences and during conversational speech.

SUMMARY OF HYPERKINETIC DYSARTHRIA

- Hyperkinetic dysarthria is actually a collection of separate dysarthrias, each associated with one of the hyperkinetic movement disorders. For example, there is the hyperkinetic dysarthria of chorea and the hyperkinetic dysarthria of dystonia. In both cases, the dysarthria is caused by involuntary movements that interfere with voluntary attempts at speech. However, because the involuntary movement patterns of the various hyperkinetic movement disorders are different, the effects of each disorder on speech production are different.

- Many, but not all, of the hyperkinetic movement disorders are associated with damage to the basal ganglia. Some of the disorders have no known cause, such as Tourette syndrome and organic tremor.

- The speech characteristics of hyperkinetic dysarthria vary according to which movement disorder is disturbing speech production.
- The most common treatment for hyperkinetic dysarthria is drug based. However, certain behaviorally based treatment procedures have been found to help some individuals with hyperkinetic dysarthria.

STUDY QUESTIONS

1. Define hyperkinetic dysarthria in your own words.
2. Why is it appropriate to describe hyperkinetic dysarthria as actually being a collection of separate dysarthrias?
3. What is one reason why the function of the basal ganglia not well understood?
4. How are the involuntary movements of chorea different from those of dystonia?
5. What are the symptoms of Huntington's disease?
6. Why do individuals with chorea sometimes have voice stoppages, unexpected inhalations, and sudden exhalations?
7. Describe fully the cause of tic disorders.
8. What is the most common hyperkinetic movement disorder?
9. What are sensory tricks; with which hyperkinetic movement disorder are they most closely associated?
10. How are most hyperkinetic movement disorders treated?

C H A P T E R

10

Mixed Dysarthria

DEFINITIONS OF MIXED DYSARTHRIA

Mixed dysarthria can occur when neurological damage extends into two or more parts of the motor system. As Duffy's following 1995 quote shows, the speech characteristics of mixed dysarthria are a combination of the characteristics found in the single (or pure) dysarthrias. The location and extent of the neurological damage determines which characteristics of the pure dysarthrias appear in a particular diagnosis of mixed dysarthria. Dworkin's quote indicates that various types of neurological damage can cause this dysarthria.

> "A mixed dysarthria . . . [is] a combination of two or more of the pure [dysarthria] types." (Duffy, 1995, p. 234)

> "Disease, illness, or injuries that cause diffuse neurologic damage may produce mixed forms of dysarthria in which a patient may present with speech and neuromuscular signs and symptoms characteristic of two or more types of the [pure] . . . dysarthrias." (Dworkin, 1991, p. 13)

NEUROLOGICAL BASIS OF MIXED DYSARTHRIA

Prior chapters of this book each examined one of the pure dysarthrias. A pure dysarthria is one in which a patient's neurological damage is restricted to a single anatomical portion of the motor system. For example, pure flaccid dysarthria occurs when the neurological damage is confined to the lower motor neurons. In other words, the damage does not extend to the upper motor neurons, cerebellum, basal ganglia, or other portions of the nervous system. The damage only affects the lower motor neurons. Similarly, in pure ataxic dysarthria, the neurological damage is confined to the cerebellum or the cerebellar control circuits. It does not extend to the lower motor neurons, the cerebral hemispheres, or other areas of the nervous system.

Realistically, however, the neurological damage resulting from strokes, head injuries, degenerative and infectious diseases, and tumors often crosses anatomical boundaries and affects various components of the motor system simultaneously. For instance, it is not unusual for a single brainstem stroke to affect both upper and lower motor neurons, because portions of these neurons are located in the brainstem. (Upper motor neurons course down through the brainstem to synapse with the lower motor neurons in the cranial and spinal nerves; lower motor neurons in the cranial nerves have their cell bodies inside the brainstem.) Consequently, it is very possible that both upper and lower motor neurons can be damaged when a stroke interrupts the flow of blood to a certain part of the brainstem. Assuming that a brainstem stroke causes bilateral damage to the pyramidal and extrapyramidal upper motor neurons *and* damages the lower motor neurons in the cranial nerves used for speech production, the result will probably be a co-occurrence of flaccid and spastic dysarthria. Such a co-occurrence of two pure dysarthrias is a mixed dysarthria. In this example, it would be described as a flaccid-spastic mixed dysarthria.

An individual with mixed dysarthria will demonstrate at least some of the speech characteristics of two or more of the pure dysarthrias. In the example of flaccid-spastic mixed dysarthria, the individual's speech might show evidence of hypernasality and nasal emission (the flaccid dysarthria component), a strained-strangled voice quality from hyperadduction of the vocal folds (the spastic component), and imprecise consonants (a characteristic that is common to both flaccid and spastic dysarthria). All three of these characteristics would be evident simultaneously in the individual's speech. The hypernasality and nasal emission could be the result of damage to the lower motor neurons of the vagus cranial nerve. The strained-strangled voice quality would be caused by bilateral damage to the upper motor neurons of the extrapyramidal system. The imprecise consonants would most likely be the combined result of lower and upper motor neuron damage.

Nearly any combination of the pure dysarthrias can appear in a mixed dysarthria, depending on the severity and extent of the neurological damage (Darley et al., 1975). As mentioned, a brainstem stroke can cause a flaccid-spastic mixed dysarthria because this is an area of the brain where the lower and upper motor neurons are in close proximity to each other. Another example of mixed dysarthria might be an individual who experiences a traumatic head injury with damage to both the cerebellum and various cranial nerves. The result could be ataxic-flaccid mixed dysarthria. A further example might be a patient with parkinsonism who has a right hemisphere stroke, causing hypokinetic-unilateral upper motor neuron mixed dysarthria. Lastly, it might be possible that a patient with Huntington's disease develops Guillain-Barré syndrome, resulting in hyperkinetic-flaccid mixed dysarthria. Although these examples may seem fanciful, mixed dysarthria is actually quite common. In fact, Duffy (1995) stated that clinicians see more cases of mixed dysarthria than any single pure dysarthria and indicated that mixed dysarthria accounted for 34.7% of all the dysarthrias seen at the Mayo Clinic during a 3-year period.

Not only can mixed dysarthria be composed of many different combinations of the pure dysarthrias; the relative prominence of each dysarthria type within a mixed dysarthria can vary significantly from individual to individual. In many instances of mixed dysarthria, one of the dysarthric components will be much more noticeable than the other(s). For example, in a flaccid-spastic mixed dysarthria, the flaccid component (perhaps nasal emission) might be much more evident to a listener than the spastic component (perhaps a strained-strangled voice quality). It also is possible, however, for each component of a mixed dysarthria to appear more or less equal in prominence. In this instance, using the example of flaccid-spastic mixed dysarthria, the listener would judge the nasal emission and the strained-strangled voice quality to be contributing equally to the dysarthric quality of the speaker's speech.

The relative prominence of one dysarthric characteristic over another is usually the result of the severity and extent of the neurological damage. When the severity is distributed equally over the affected portions of the motor system, the resulting characteristics of the mixed dysarthria may be equally evident to a listener. However, when one part of the motor system is more seriously affected than the other, the dysarthric component associated with the more severely damaged portion usually will be more apparent to a listener.

It also is important to note that the relative prominence of one dysarthric component over another can change over time. For example, amyotrophic lateral sclerosis (ALS) is a progressive motor neuron disease that often first affects lower motor neurons, which results in flaccid dysarthria. As the disease progresses, however, it eventually begins to affect upper motor neurons as well, causing a flaccid-spastic mixed dysarthria. Initially, in this mixed dysarthria, the flaccid components are more noticeable than the spastic components. In time, however, the upper motor neuron damage usually becomes equal to that of the lower motor neurons. At this stage, the spastic component of the dysarthria may be as evident as the flaccid. ALS is discussed in greater detail later in this chapter.

Both beginning and experienced clinicians often find it difficult to make a correct diagnosis for mixed dysarthria. This may be because of the multiple speech deficits that are usually present in mixed dysarthria, compared to a pure dysarthria. Although often challenging, it is still important to diagnose mixed dysarthria as accurately as possible. A precise diagnosis can provide helpful information about a patient's disorder. To illustrate this, Duffy (1995) used the example of a patient with a diagnosis of Parkinson's disease that presented a hypokinetic-ataxic mixed dysarthria. The presence of this mixed dysarthria indicated one of two possibilities about the diagnosis of Parkinson's disease: Either the diagnosis was incorrect or the patient had something in addition to Parkinson's disease. This is because ataxic dysarthria is not a symptom of Parkinson's disease. The presence of ataxic dysarthria in the patient's speech indicated that further diagnostic work was needed. Situations such as this can occur frequently and demonstrate the value of having a good understanding of all the dysarthrias.

ETIOLOGIES OF MIXED DYSARTHRIA

Many disorders can cause mixed dysarthria. Some of these include single or multiple strokes, brain tumors, traumatic head injuries, degenerative diseases, infectious diseases, and others. In fact, any disorder that can damage two or more parts of the motor system has the potential to cause mixed dysarthria. Because so many conditions have this potential, a complete listing of all the disorders and combinations of disorders that can lead to this dysarthria would be very long indeed. Accordingly, the following paragraphs concentrate on a several specific diseases that typically have mixed dysarthria as a prominent symptom. The reader is reminded, however, that numerous other conditions can cause mixed dysarthria in addition to those discussed here.

Multiple Sclerosis

Multiple sclerosis (MS) is a progressive disease in which the myelin covering of axons degenerates. MS is the most common of the demyelinating diseases. It occurs in about 100 per 100,000 of the population in the United States and United Kingdom. MS usually first appears when individuals are in their 30s. Women are affected more frequently than men are by a ratio of 1.7 to 1 (Wiederholt, 1995). Interestingly, MS is most prevalent in individuals who live in cold and temperate areas. It is uncommon among those living in the tropics.

The etiology of MS is unknown, but some evidence suggests that it may be an immunological disorder that is triggered by a virus. The myelin degeneration of MS usually appears first as small points of inflammation. Eventually, the inflammation can increase in severity until the myelin and cells that produce it (oligodendrocytes) are destroyed. The amount of affected myelin along the length of an axon can range from only a millimeter to a few centimeters. It is important to note that MS does not directly damage the axon. It remains intact, but the destruction of the protective myelin affects its function by slowing or stopping its ability to conduct neural impulses.

MS may affect myelin almost anywhere in the CNS. Not only can MS affect the myelin-rich white matter areas of the CNS; it also can attack myelin-covered gray matter in the CNS. Consequently, MS can occur in the brainstem, cerebellum, cerebral hemispheres, and spinal cord. Some patients have symptoms that suggest focal MS lesions in only one area of the brain. For example, a patient's main symptoms might be ataxic in nature, suggesting a focal cerebellar lesion. In contrast, other patients can demonstrate a diffuse collection of symptoms, indicating widespread MS lesions in multiple areas of the CNS.

The symptoms of MS are diverse. It often is mentioned in medical textbooks that no two patients with MS have exactly the same symptoms. Nevertheless, the general symptoms of MS can be grouped into several broad categories. Visual disturbances are among the most common complaints of individuals with this disease. These disturbances include double vision (diplopia), impairment of color perception, decreased visual acuity, and impaired central vision (central scotoma). The motor disturbances of MS include chronic feelings of tiredness; weakness in the limbs, particularly in the legs; painful spasticity in the extremities, again particularly in the legs; disturbances of sphincter muscle control; and dysarthria. The sensory disturbances include numbness, burning sensations, itching, and tingling. Depression also is a common complaint of patients with MS, and a mild dementia may be noted in some advanced cases of the disease.

The course of MS varies significantly from patient to patient. Wiederholt (1995) described four different ways in which MS progresses:

- About 40% of patients go through relapsing and remitting occurrences of their symptoms during the early stages of the disease. After several years, however, this changes, and the patients begin a slow but steady progression of increasingly more significant symptoms.
- About 20% to 30% of patients maintain a relapsing and remitting course of MS for the duration of their lives. They never experience a steadily progressive increase in symptoms.
- About 10% to 20% of patients have a steady progression of symptoms from the very outset of the disease.
- About 20% of patients experience only one or two relapsing and remitting occurrences of symptoms during their lifetimes. They are otherwise unaffected by the disease.

Speech Characteristics of Multiple Sclerosis

Although MS can cause many types of dysarthria, most individuals with this disease do not demonstrate obvious motor speech deficits. In their study of 168 individuals with MS, Darley, Brown, and Goldstein (1972) found that 59% of their subjects had no evidence of dysarthria, as would be judged by an average listener. Moreover, 28% had an overall deviant speech rating of only "minimal." Taken as a whole, these data indicate that 87% of the subjects with MS had adequate speech or only minor speech deficits. Nonetheless, some of the subjects who were judged to have essentially normal speech still demonstrated a few problems, primarily in controlling the loudness of their voice and in producing a clear phonation. Darley et al. (1972) summarized their findings by stating that the most prominent speech errors in individuals with MS are deficits of loudness control, harshness, and impaired articulation. Table 10–1 lists all the speech deficits noted in the Darley et al. study. Based on the results of this and other studies, Duffy (1995) suggested that ataxic and spastic dysarthria are the two most common pure dysarthrias found in MS, and ataxic-spastic is the most common mixed dysarthria associated with this disease. Duffy also mentioned that MS has the potential to cause any of the pure dysarthrias or any combination of the mixed dysarthrias. Given that MS can affect so many differ-

Table 10–1. The 10 Most Common Speech Production Errors in Individuals With Multiple Sclerosis

Rank	Speech Production Errors
1	Impaired loudness control
2	Harsh voice quality
3	Imprecise articulation
4	Impaired emphasis (scanning speech)
5	Decreased vital capacity
6	Hypernasality
7	Inappropriate pitch level
8	Breathiness
9	Increased breathing rate
10	Sudden articulatory breakdowns

Source: From "Dysarthria in Multiple Sclerosis," by F. L. Darley, J. R. Brown, and N. P. Goldstein, 1972, *Journal of Speech and Hearing Research, 15*, p. 236. Copyright 1972 by American Speech-Language-Hearing Association. Reprinted with permission.

ent portions of the nervous system, it should not be surprising that there can be numerous types of dysarthria associated with it.

Multisystems Atrophy

Multisystems atrophy is another progressive condition that can cause mixed dysarthria. It is not a single disorder, however. Multisystems atrophy actually is a collective term for a group of degenerative disorders, many of which include parkinsonian symptoms. Although there are many disorders classified under the multisystems umbrella, only three are discussed in this textbook.

Shy-Drager Syndrome

Shy-Drager syndrome is a degenerative neurological disease that primarily affects neurons in the brainstem, basal ganglia, and autonomic nervous system. It usually first appears in middle age and progresses slowly. It is often fatal several years after its onset. Patients with Shy-Drager syndrome do not develop dementia. Its cause is unknown.

Parkinsonlike symptoms are among the many signs of this syndrome. Bradykinesia, akinesia, and rigidity can all be present, but tremor is often absent or may be greatly reduced in intensity, compared to the other forms of parkinsonism. Unfortunately, l-dopa and other antiparkinson drugs are ineffective in treating the parkinsonian symptoms of this disorder. Some of the other symptoms of Shy-Drager syndrome include mild spasticity in the limbs, face, or neck, which is caused by bilateral degeneration of upper motor neurons. Damage to the autonomic nervous system can result in problems in regulating blood pressure, impotence, bowel and bladder dysfunction, and poor pupillary reaction to light. This syndrome also can affect the cerebellum or its control circuits and cause signs of ataxia.

Several combinations of mixed dysarthria have been noted in cases of Shy-Drager syndrome (Linebaugh, 1979). The three most common are spastic-ataxic-hypokinetic, hypokinetic-ataxic, and ataxic-spastic mixed dysarthria. These combinations of dysarthria reflect neurological degeneration in the basal ganglia, upper motor neurons, and cerebellum.

Progressive Supranuclear Palsy

A second multisystems degenerative disorder is known as progressive supranuclear palsy. This is a rare disease with a prevalence of 1.4 per

100,000 of the population (Warlow, 1991). Progressive supranuclear palsy causes the degeneration of neurons in the brainstem, basal ganglia, and cerebellum. It often appears in late middle age and follows a steadily progressive course. The cause of progressive supranuclear palsy is unknown, and it is usually fatal after several years. The most characteristic symptom is the gradual restriction of voluntary eye movements, which makes it difficult for these patients to walk down stairs, read, or notice objects in their peripheral vision. Problems with walking and neck rigidity are the most obvious parkinsonian symptoms of this disease, but a generalized rigidity can develop as the disease progresses. Bilateral upper motor neuron involvement can result in mild spasticity of the limbs, face, or neck. Other symptoms of progressive supranuclear palsy include dementia, dysphagia, involuntary closing of the eyelid (blepharospasm), and dysarthria.

Several types of dysarthria are associated with progressive supranuclear palsy. In summarizing the findings of several studies, Duffy (1995) stated that hypokinetic, spastic, or mixed hypokinetic-spastic dysarthria are the most common dysarthrias in this disease. In addition, he reported that ataxic dysarthria also can be present in progressive supranuclear palsy, frequently in conjunction with either hypokinetic or spastic dysarthria.

Olivopontocerebellar Atrophy

The final multisystems atrophy disorder discussed is olivopontocerebellar atrophy. This disorder causes the gradual deterioration of neurons in the inferior olivary nucleus, pons, and cerebellum. The inferior olivary nucleus is a collection of neuron cell bodies in the brainstem near the cerebellar peduncles.

Olivopontocerebellar atrophy is a rare disease, and the cause is unknown. Familial links have been clearly established in some cases. The onset of this disorder usually occurs when individuals are in their 30s or 40s. The symptoms include ataxic disturbances of balance, uncoordinated movements of the arms and legs, tremor, numbness in the extremities, muscle spasms, problems with bowel and bladder control, and dysarthria. Involuntary choreic movements and mild dementia have been noted in some individuals. There is no cure for olivopontocerebellar atrophy; it progresses quite slowly and leads to death about 20 years after the first onset of symptoms.

Because of the different areas of the brain affected by this disease, the dysarthria associated with it is most frequently of the mixed type. It may have components of ataxic, spastic, flaccid, or hypokinetic dysarthria (Duffy, 1995), although little research has been conducted into the speech deficits of this disorder.

Amyotrophic Lateral Sclerosis

Amyotrophic lateral sclerosis (ALS) is a disease that results in the progressive degeneration of motor neurons. The cause of ALS is unknown. It occurs in about 1.5 per 100,000 of the population worldwide. Although it can develop in individuals as young as 20 or as old as 90, the median age of onset is 65 years (Wiederholt, 1995). Males are affected more frequently than females by a ratio of 1.5 to 1. About 5% of individuals with ALS have a close relative who also has had the disease (Warlow, 1991). In nearly all cases, ALS is relentlessly progressive and is fatal within the first few months or years after onset, although some individuals survive for many years longer than this. Most patients die from complications of pneumonia and respiratory failure.

ALS can affect motor neurons in any of four areas of the motor system. It may occur (a) in the spinal nerves at the point where they join the spinal cord (the anterior horn cells of the spinal cord), (b) in the cranial nerves where they join the brainstem (the cranial nerve nuclei), (c) in the upper motor neurons of the corticospinal tracts, and (d) in the upper motor neurons of the corticobulbar tracts. Depending on which motor neurons are affected first, patients with ALS *initially* may demonstrate one of four possible clusters of symptoms.

- Patients with spinal nerve involvement will demonstrate weakness in their arms and legs, loss of muscle tone, muscle atrophy, and decreased reflexes.
- Patients with cranial nerve involvement will demonstrate flaccid dysarthria, a reduced gag reflex, tongue atrophy, dysphagia, and facial and oral weakness.
- Patients with involvement of the upper motor neurons of the corticospinal tract will demonstrate weakness and spasticity in the arms and legs, increased reflexes, and painful muscle cramps in the extremities.
- Patients with involvement of the upper motor neurons of the corticobulbar tract will demonstrate spastic dysarthria, hyperactive gag reflexes, facial and oral weakness, and dysphagia.

As mentioned, early in the course of ALS only one or two of the motor neuron groups will be affected, but as the disease progresses, all four groups are likely to be involved. In the end stages of ALS, weakness and muscle atrophy prevents nearly all attempts at movement. Dementia is not a symptom of this disease; patients with ALS maintain their cognitive abilities throughout the course of the disease. Their bodily sensations, eye movements, and bladder control remain essentially intact as well.

Speech Characteristics of Amyotrophic Lateral Sclerosis

The type of dysarthria that appears in individuals with ALS depends on which motor neurons are affected by the disorder. Those with lower motor neuron involvement will demonstrate flaccid dysarthria. Conversely, those predominantly with upper motor neuron involvement will demonstrate spastic dysarthria. When the disease progresses to the point where both upper and lower motor neurons are affected, patients with ALS will demonstrate flaccid-spastic mixed dysarthria. The pure dysarthrias probably will be present only in the disease's initial, mild stages. The mixed dysarthria condition will predominate throughout most of the disorder.

In their study of 30 subjects with ALS, Darley et al. (1969a, 1969b) found that the subjects' speech errors reflected the combined characteristics of flaccid and spastic dysarthria. The three most prominent errors in their subjects' speech were imprecise consonants, hypernasality, and harsh vocal quality. The ranking of 10 speech characteristics of their subjects with ALS is presented in Table 10–2.

However, a simple ranking of speech errors does not accurately express the devastating effects of ALS on speech production. Perhaps Darley et al. (1975) presented the best description of the speech of an individual with ALS as they concluded their discussion of this disorder:

> The speech gestalt distinctive of ALS, then, consists of grossly defective articulation of both consonants and vowels, often rendering the speech unintelligible; laborious, extremely slow production of words in very short phrases; marked hypernasality coupled with severe harshness and strained-strangled squeezing out of low-pitched tones; and complete disruption of prosody, with monotony suppressing meaningfulness and intervals between words and phrases becoming excessive. (p. 235)

Wilson's Disease

Wilson's disease is another disorder that can cause a mixed dysarthria. It is a very rare hereditary disease that prevents the normal metabolism

Table 10–2. The 10 Most Common Speech Production Errors in 30 Individuals With Amyotrophic Lateral Sclerosis

Rank	Speech Production Errors
1	Imprecise consonants
2	Hypernasality
3	Harsh voice quality
4	Slow rate
5	Monopitch
6	Short phrases
7	Distorted vowels
8	Low Pitch
9	Monoloudness
10	Excess and equal stress

Source: From "Clusters of Diagnostic Patterns of Dysarthria," by F. L. Darley, A. E. Aronson, and J. R. Brown, 1969, *Journal of Speech and Hearing Research, 12*, p. 254. Copyright 1969 by American Speech-Language-Hearing Association. Adapted with permission.

of dietary copper. Although small amounts of copper are a necessary nutritional mineral, individuals with Wilson's disease cannot metabolize it properly. Instead of being excreted, excessive amounts of copper are deposited in the corneas of the eyes, kidneys, liver, and brain (especially in the basal ganglia). The buildup of copper in these organs produces a unique collection of cognitive, motor, and psychiatric symptoms. The first signs of Wilson's disease usually appear when the affected individuals are in their teens or twenties. The early symptoms include clumsiness, mild decreases in cognitive abilities, and subtle personality changes. The later symptoms include rigidity, bradykinesia, tremor, limb ataxia, dementia, dysphagia, and dysarthria. Dystonic and choreic movements have also been observed in cases of Wilson's disease. The psychiatric symptoms of this disorder can be significant. These include emotional lability, severe depression, mania, and behaviors having schizophrenic characteristics (Lechtenberg, 1982). Incidentally, the copper deposited in the eye creates a brown-colored ring around the edges of the cornea that can be seen under certain lighting conditions.

Fortunately, effective treatments are available for nearly all individuals with this disease. The most common treatment is oral dosages of penicillamine. This drug is able to reduce the copper deposits in the body and often leads to dramatic improvements in all symptoms. However, permanent damage can occur if the treatment is not initiated quickly enough. If left untreated, Wilson's disease can be fatal within 2 or 3 years after the first appearance of symptoms. In untreated cases, death usually occurs from liver failure.

Speech Characteristics of Wilson's Disease

Ever since Wilson disease was first documented, numerous researchers have commented that dysarthria is a common feature of this disorder (Darley et al., 1975). In fact, dysarthria may one of the earliest signs of Wilson's disease. Berry, Darley, Aronson, and Goldstein (1974) conducted the most extensive study of the dysarthria associated with this disease. They analyzed the speech of 20 subjects with Wilson's disease. The results showed that reduced stress, monopitch, and monoloudness were the three most prominent speech errors in the subjects. The researchers noted that hypokinetic dysarthria is one of the most noticeable dysarthrias in Wilson's disease. The results also revealed speech errors that were characteristic of ataxic and spastic dysarthria. Overall, the study found that many individuals with Wilson's disease demonstrate an ataxic-spastic-hypokinetic mixed dysarthria, with any one of these three components possibly being more prominent than the others. Furthermore, it was noted that any of these components might appear alone in some individuals with Wilson's disease, reflecting a pure rather than a mixed dysarthria. The ranking of speech errors in this study is presented in Table 10–3.

In an interesting addendum to this study, Berry, Aronson, Darley, and Goldstein (1974) followed 10 subjects with Wilson's disease during 3 years of treatment with low copper diets and penicillamine. The researchers obtained pretreatment and posttreatment measures of speech production to measure any changes in the subjects' dysarthria during the treatment period. Although the subjects still had some dysarthric qualities in their speech at the end of the treatment period, there were significant improvements in nearly all areas of speech production, especially intelligibility. Overall, the improvements were remarkable. Duffy (1995) suggested that changes in speech during the medical treatment of Wilsons disease could serve as an indicator of treatment effectiveness.

Friedreich's Ataxia

Friedreich's ataxia is an inherited, progressive disorder that causes neuron degeneration in the cerebellum, brainstem, and spinal cord (in

Table 10–3. The 10 Most Common Speech Production Errors in 20 Individuals With Wilson's Disease

Rank	Speech Production Errors
1	Reduced Stress
2	Monopitch
3	Monoloudness
4	Imprecise consonants
5	Slow rate
6	Excess and equal stress
7	Low pitch
8	Irregular articulatory breakdowns
9	Hypernasality
10	Inappropriate silences

Source: From "Dysarthria in Wilson's disease," by W. R. Berry, F. L. Darley, A. E. Aronson, and N. P. Goldstein, 1974, *Journal of Speech and Hearing Research, 17*, p. 175. Copyright 1974 by American Speech-Language-Hearing Association. Reprinted with permission.

particular). As mentioned briefly in Chapter 7, this is a rare disorder that first becomes evident when individuals are in their 20s. It is untreatable and usually is fatal within 10 to 15 years after the initial appearance of the symptoms. Death is often the result of heart failure or coma. The early symptoms of Friedreich's ataxia are unsteadiness and clumsiness, with ataxia being present in the movements of the arms and legs (Warlow, 1991). Mild dysarthria also may be an early symptom. As the disorder progresses, weakness and muscle atrophy becomes evident in the arms and legs. Visual deficits and sensorineural hearing loss also can occur in the later stages. Some individuals with Friedreich's ataxia eventually develop dementia.

Although Friedreich's ataxia can cause pure ataxic dysarthria, mixed dysarthria is also common. Joanette and Dudley (1980) found what appeared to be an ataxic-spastic mixed dysarthria in their 22 patients with this disorder. In his discussion of the speech pathology of Friedreich's ataxia, Duffy (1995) suggested that ataxic dysarthria is the most common dysarthria associated with this disease, but other types may be present, especially spastic dysarthria. In addition, he concluded that ataxic-spastic mixed dysarthria is probably the most prevalent of the mixed dysarthrias in this disorder.

TREATMENT OF MIXED DYSARTHRIA

Without doubt, treating mixed dysarthria can be a challenge. There may be so many speech errors that many clinicians are not sure where to start. The general rule in treating mixed dysarthria is to first treat the component that is most severely affecting speech production. As an illustration of this, imagine a patient with flaccid-ataxic mixed dysarthria where the flaccid characteristics are impairing intelligibility more noticeably than the ataxic characteristics. The first steps of treatment would concentrate on the flaccid elements. Once they had been addressed sufficiently, treatment could then shift to the ataxic characteristics of the dysarthria. However, this is only a general treatment principle, and there will be situations where it will not be particularly helpful, such as when the various elements of a mixed dysarthria are contributing equally to the patient's speech production difficulties.

When the elements of a mixed dysarthria are equally affecting speech production, Dworkin (1991) suggested that treatment be sequenced according to which of the components of speech production (i.e., respiration, articulation, phonation, resonation, and prosody) are being affected most by the dysarthria. He recommended that errors of respiration be treated first, then resonation, followed by phonation, then articulation, and lastly prosody. Thus, if a patient with mixed dysarthria is demonstrating equal measures of monopitch, imprecise consonants, and hypernasality, the recommended treatment sequence would be resonation first, articulation second, and prosody third.

The reason for completing the treatments in this order is based on how the different components of speech support each other. For example, respiration is addressed first because it is the foundation for all other speech components. Without adequate respiratory support, resonation, phonation, articulation, and prosody are all impaired to one degree or another. For instance, it would be difficult to treat a phonatory problem if a patient's respiration was too weak to create adequate phonation. Likewise, it would impossible to treat many prosodic problems if deficits of resonation, articulation, and so forth had not been addressed beforehand.

In a situation where there is more than one problem within a single component of speech production, treatment usually should address the most severe problem first. An example of this is a patient who has more than one deficit of prosody, perhaps someone who has very prolonged intervals between syllables and moderately excessive loudness variations. Because both of these are prosodic errors, Dworkin's recommended treatment sequence does not apply. Nevertheless, the most likely treatment choice would be to treat the error that is most affecting the patient's prosody. If the clinician makes the judgment that the prolonged syllable interval is the more serious problem, treatment would concentrate on it first. However, this treatment choice assumes that deficits of respiration, resonation, phonation, or articulation have been ruled out as the cause of the prosodic problems.

Naturally, there will be special exceptions to this rule of treating the most severe error first. For example, a patient might have a strong preference for what needs to be treated initially; perhaps it is something that is personally very annoying or frustrating. Maybe a patient's attention or memory deficit makes working on a particular type of speech production error extremely difficult, but he or she is able to make progress on another type of speech error. In situations such as these, it may be appropriate to choose the less severe speech production deficit for treatment, based on the unique circumstances that might be present.

Augmentative Communication for Patients with ALS

In many of the progressive neurological disorders discussed in this chapter, the patient will reach the point where intelligible verbal communication is no longer possible. This will occur for about 75% of individuals with ALS (Saunders, Walsh, & Smith, 1981) and about 4% of individuals with MS (Beukelman, Kraft, & Freal, 1985). When verbal speech becomes impossible, the most appropriate option is some type of augmentative communication. Beukelman and Mirenda (1998) described five communicative stages through which a patient with ALS will pass as the disease progresses. For each stage, they discussed the responsibilities of speech-language pathologists working with a person with ALS. Clinicians should remember that there is no typical timetable for when a given patient will move from one stage to another. As mentioned earlier, the full progression of ALS is quite variable, ranging from months to decades. Some patients with ALS will spend weeks or months at one of these stages; others will spend years.

1. No Detectable Speech Disorder

During this first stage, patients and families can be given general facts about the communication deficits associated with ALS. Because of the high likelihood that augmentative communication will be needed eventually, patients should start learning the basics of these systems in this early stage of the disease. For example, patients should learn what communication methods are available and any special features that make them unique. However, Beukelman and Mirenda cautioned that at this first stage, it might be premature and counterproductive to give too many details about the challenges augmentative communication ultimately will present to a patient with ALS.

2. Obvious Speech Disorder With Intelligible Speech

In this second stage, patients begin to demonstrate speech errors that most listeners can easily detect, but their intelligibility remains high. Beukelman and Mirenda suggested that speech pathologists should become more actively involved in advising a patient and family on how to maximize the intelligibility of the patient's speech. For example, family members are told about avoiding conversation in noisy settings and how to ensure that listeners understand when a topic of conversation is being changed. It also may be appropriate for a patient to be introduced to voice amplification at this time, if he or she will be speaking in conversational groups. The preliminary steps of assessing and choosing augmentative communication systems should be started at this stage.

3. Reduction in Speech Intelligibility

When patients reach this point, their dysarthria is clearly interfering with speech intelligibility. Many of the treatments for flaccid or spastic dysarthria that were presented in Chapters 5 and 6 can help increase or maintain a patient's intelligibility, at least temporarily. For example, speaking with a more open-position mouth, breath group duration, palatal lift, reduced rate of speech, and exaggerating consonants might be appropriate treatments for a patient's dysarthric deficits. Beukelman and Mirenda also recommended that augmentative communication systems be in place for patients in this third stage of the disease.

4. Residual Natural Speech and Augmentative Communication

In this fourth stage, patients with ALS rely heavily on augmentative communication to supplement their residual intelligible speech. In fact, Beukelman and Mirenda stated that augmentative communication now becomes the primary method of communication. At this stage, the speech pathologist is involved in assessing the adequacy of the augmentative communication systems, such as determining if a system is the best match for a patient's remaining motor capabilities or if the physical position of a system maximizes the patient's ability to use it.

Speech pathologists also will be involved in training family members and friends on the best methods of communicating with someone who is using an augmentative communication device.

5. Loss of Useful Speech

At this final stage, patients with ALS have lost nearly all of their intelligible speech and depend almost exclusively on augmentative communication systems to make their wants and needs known. In addition to using sophisticated electronic devices, Beukelman and Mirenda recommended that a collection of low-tech augmentative procedures also be used to maximize a patient's ability to communicate. These include simple yes/no communication methods, eye-pointing techniques, and eye blinks.

SUMMARY OF MIXED DYSARTHRIA

- Mixed dysarthria can occur when damage involves more than one portion of the motor system. For example, when the lower motor neurons and the cerebellum are damaged, the result can be a flaccid-ataxic mixed dysarthria.
- Depending on the extent and location of the neurological damage, any combination of the pure dysarthrias can be the components of a mixed dysarthria.
- Within a mixed dysarthria, it is possible for one of the components to be more noticeable than the other(s).
- There are many conditions that can cause mixed dysarthria. Head injury, stroke, brain tumor, and numerous degenerative or infectious diseases are all possible etiologies of mixed dysarthria.
- Amyotrophic lateral sclerosis and multiple sclerosis are the two most well known degenerative disorders that can cause mixed dysarthria.
- The general treatment sequence for mixed dysarthria is to first treat the portion that is contributing most to a patient's speech production deficits.
- If the elements of a mixed dysarthria are contributing equally to the patient's problems, Dworkin (1991) recommended treating the components of speech production in the sequence: (a) respiration, (b) resonation, (c) phonation, (d) articulation, and finally (e) prosody.

STUDY QUESTIONS

1. Define mixed dysarthria in your own words.
2. Describe how multiple strokes could lead to a mixed dysarthria.
3. Damage to which anatomical sites would be likely to cause an ataxic-hypokinetic-spastic mixed dysarthria?
4. Why do many clinicians find mixed dysarthria to be a challenge to diagnose?
5. Why can multiple sclerosis result in almost any type of dysarthria?
6. What are the three multisystems atrophy disorders that were discussed in this chapter, and what type of dysarthria can they cause?
7. Describe the four areas of the motor system that can be affected by amyotrophic lateral sclerosis?
8. What type of mixed dysarthria is most associated with the latter stages of amyotrophic lateral sclerosis?
9. What is the cause of Wilson's disease?
10. What treatment sequence does Dworkin recommend when all components of a mixed dysarthria are contributing equally to a patient's speech production errors?

C H A P T E R

11

Apraxia of Speech

DEFINITIONS OF APRAXIA OF SPEECH

The following two definitions of apraxia of speech highlight a few of the major characteristics of this disorder. They mention that it is a problem with sequencing the movements needed to produce speech and that apraxic speech errors are inconsistent. The variable nature of apraxic speech errors is one of the characteristics that differentiates this disorder from dysarthria, which typically results in more consistent errors. Miller's definition also indicates that individuals with apraxia of speech often struggle to find the correct articulatory positions needed to produce phonemes accurately.

> An articulatory disorder resulting from impairment, as a result of brain damage, of the capacity to program the positioning of speech musculature and the sequencing of muscle movements for the volitional production of phonemes. No significant weakness, slowness, or incoordination in reflex and automatic acts. Prosodic alterations may be associated with the articulatory problem, perhaps in compensation for it. (Darley, 1969)

> [Individuals with apraxia of speech] can be said to have difficulty in consistently realizing speech sounds. Sometimes they say a sound or word correctly, and other times they do not. Speakers can often be seen to be struggling to get the right placements of lips, tongue and so on, which are eluding them even though they can produce the same sound or word perfectly normally another time. (Miller, 1986, p. 99)

OVERVIEW OF THE APRAXIAS

This chapter examines a motor speech disorder known as apraxia of speech. Like the dysarthrias, apraxia of speech is a neurological deficit in the production of speech sounds. However, unlike the dysarthrias, the errors in apraxia of speech are not caused by muscle weakness, abnormal muscle tone, reduced range of movement, or decreased muscle steadiness. Rather, the errors in this disorder are caused by a deficit in the ability to accurately sequence the movements needed to produce speech sounds.

As was mentioned in Chapter 1, the term *apraxia* comes from the Greek word *praxis*, which means "performance of action." Apraxia literally means "without action." In fact, it is probably more accurate to describe this disorder as dyspraxia (which means, "disordered action") because, strictly speaking, individuals with apraxia of speech are not without movement. They can move their tongue, lips, velum, and so forth. Their problem is with the sequencing of movements needed to produce speech. But because apraxia has become such a common word for describing this disorder, it is the one that is used in this chapter.

There are several types of apraxia, of which apraxia of speech is only one of the subcategories. The two main types of apraxia are ideational apraxia and ideomotor apraxia. **Ideational apraxia** is the inability to make use of an object or gesture because the individual has lost the knowledge (or idea) of the object's or gesture's function. In other words, individuals with ideational apraxia cannot make proper use of an object or gesture because they no longer know its purpose. A head-injured patient of Luria's (1972) gave a good example of ideational apraxia when describing an event that occurred in a hospital:

> I was lying in bed and needed a nurse. How was I to get her to come over? All of a sudden I remembered you can beckon to someone and so I tried to beckon to the nurse—that is, move my left hand lightly back and forth. But she walked right on by and paid no attention to my gesturing. I realized then that I'd completely forgotten how to beckon to someone. It appeared I'd even forgotten how to gesture with my hands so that someone could understand what I meant. (p. 45)

Ideational apraxia is an uncommon disorder that usually seems to result from damage to the left parietal lobe. It often goes undetected, because its symptoms can be masked so easily by an accompanying disorder such as aphasia. It also is difficult to detect because it often resolves quickly when caused by a stroke (Miller, 1986).

The second main type of apraxia is **ideomotor apraxia**. In contrast to ideational apraxia, which is a disturbance in the *conception* of an object or gesture, ideomotor apraxia is a disturbance in the *performance* of the movements needed to use an object, make a gesture, or complete a sequence of individual movements. Apraxia of speech is one of the ideomotor apraxias. Individuals with ideomotor apraxia have not lost their knowledge of an object or gesture's function; they have a deficit in carrying out the motor plan needed to use an object or make a gesture. When asked, for example, to use a common object such as a toothbrush, an individual with ideational apraxia may demonstrate the general pattern of movements required to brush the teeth, indicating that he or she understands the purpose of the toothbrush. For instance, the individual may hold the toothbrush properly and move it toward the mouth. However, the separate movements needed to actually brush the teeth may be out of sequence. Perhaps the up and down motion of brushing the front teeth becomes the back and forth movement of brushing the molars or vice versa. The individual's attempts to revise and correct these out of sequence movements result in toothbrushing that is halting, slow, and awkward.

Ideomotor apraxia has been studied extensively since it was first described in the 1900s. Numerous characteristics of this disorder have been noted. The following is a list of the more well-known symptoms of ideomotor apraxia. It should be noted, however, that these are symptoms that are likely to be present in cases of *pure* ideomotor apraxia. When additional motor, language, or cognitive deficits accompany the apraxia, these symptoms may be masked by these other problems and will not necessarily be as evident as these descriptions might suggest.

- Ideomotor apraxia typically affects voluntary movements far more often than spontaneous or automatic movements. For example, if asked to voluntarily wave goodbye on command, an individual with ideomotor apraxia may not be able to successfully sequence the movements needed to accurately complete the action. Even if the action is complete, the overall movements may be effortful and clumsy. However, if the individual actually were leaving a social situation, the hand wave would be smooth and effortless. Another example of this might involve a movement such as a smile. An individual with ideomotor apraxia may not be able to smile promptly when asked to do so, but a moment later a spontaneous smile might appear without difficulty, if something amusing happens unexpectedly.
- Movement sequencing is easier when actually manipulating a real object compared to only pantomiming its use. For example, an individual with ideomotor apraxia will probably be more successful in showing how to drink from a cup when actually given a cup, compared to only pretending to have one.
- Completing a movement sequence is easier when given a gestural command (imitation), compared to being given a verbal command. In other words, individuals with ideomotor apraxia may not be able to round their lips when they are verbally asked to do so, but they may be successful when a clinician demonstrates the movement for them.
- The movement sequencing errors in ideomotor apraxia are often very inconsistent, even on repeated attempts at the same movement. An example of this might be when an individual with apraxia of speech tries to say a multisyllabic word. On the first attempt, an extra syllable might be added to the word. On the next attempt the added syllable may be gone, but now a phoneme substitution appears in the word. On the third

attempt, yet another type of error might occur, perhaps a severe distortion of one or more phonemes.

There are at least three subcategories of ideomotor apraxia. The first is **limb apraxia**. This is the inability to sequence the movements of the arms, legs, hands, or feet during a voluntary action, although the concept behind the action and the general motor plan appears to be accurate. The toothbrush example is an example of this type of apraxia. Limb apraxia is most often the result of left hemisphere damage. In a majority of cases, it affects both the right and left limbs, although hemiplegia may hide its effects on one side of the body. This disorder is usually assessed by having the individual pantomime a variety of well-known movements, such as hammering a nail, shaving, putting a key in a lock, and combing hair.

A second subcategory of ideomotor apraxia is **nonverbal oral apraxia**. This type of apraxia is also known as buccofacial apraxia, facial apraxia, orofacial apraxia, or lingual apraxia. As its name implies, nonverbal oral apraxia is a deficit in the ability to sequence nonverbal, voluntary movements of the tongue, lips, jaw, and other associated oral structures. The orofacial movements affected by this disorder might include protruding the tongue, whistling, biting the lower lip, and puffing out the cheeks. When asked to perform tasks such as these, an individual with this type of apraxia may grope for the correct position of the mouth, delay performing the action, only partially complete the movement, or perhaps add extra, unnecessary movements. Occasionally, some individuals with nonverbal oral apraxia have trouble performing voluntary movements that are only partially associated with the oral mechanism. For example, they may have trouble taking a deep breath when asked to do so, or they may be unable to swallow on command.

Nonverbal oral apraxia is commonly seen in individuals with left hemisphere damage, and it can often co-occur with aphasia. Although this disorder can be puzzling and even distressing to the patient, it does not affect spontaneous or reflexive orofacial movements. This means that the individual will still be able swallow while eating, breathe deeply when out of breath, smile at a joke, and make other spontaneous movements of the oral mechanism. Because individuals with this disorder usually are able to perform these important automatic oral movement without difficulty, nonverbal oral apraxia is usually thought to have little clinical significance (Wertz et al., 1991). For the speech-language pathologist, this type of apraxia is of interest primarily because it can co-occur with the third subcategory of ideomotor apraxia: apraxia of speech.

Apraxia of speech is a deficit in the ability to sequence the motor commands needed to correctly position the articulators during the voluntary production of phonemes. Because most speech is a voluntary motor task, apraxia of speech can have serious effects on a patient's ability to communicate orally. Apraxia of speech is a disorder specific to the sequencing of the movements needed to produce phonemes, and it can co-occur with limb or nonverbal oral apraxia. The distinction between nonverbal oral apraxia and apraxia of speech is evident in the names of these two disorders. Nonverbal oral apraxia is a disturbance in the sequencing of oral movements that are *unrelated to speech production*, such as licking the lips, blowing out a match, and moving the tongue from side to side. Apraxia of speech, as already stated, is a disturbance in the sequencing of the oral movements in speech production. Although it is common to have a co-occurrence of these two apraxias in the same individual, both can appear more or less separately. For example, some individuals may have apraxia of speech but not have obvious symptoms of nonverbal oral apraxia, and other individuals may have nonverbal oral apraxia but not obvious symptoms of apraxia of speech.

Apraxia of speech is usually caused by damage to the left frontal lobe, especially when the damage occurs near Broca's area. Because apraxia of speech is so often associated with damage to the left hemisphere, cases of pure apraxia of speech are actually quite rare. In the majority of cases, apraxia of speech co-occurs with Broca's aphasia. In addition, it is common for it to co-occur with unilateral upper motor neuron dysarthria as well (Duffy, 1995). The simultaneous occurrence of these disorders can make it difficult for a beginning clinician to separate the motor speech errors of apraxia from the language and articulation errors of a co-occurring aphasia and dysarthria. The remainder of this chapter is designed to make it easier for the inexperienced clinician to identify the symptoms of apraxia of speech and treat them appropriately.

NEUROLOGICAL BASIS OF APRAXIA OF SPEECH

As with so much of the central nervous system, the method by which motor commands are sequenced for speech is not well understood. This lack of understanding is a reflection of how complex the task of motor speech programming is. For instance, sequencing the motor commands of speech production require input from many different areas of the brain. The language centers provide the linguistic information that is to be spoken, including the phonemes that need to be sequenced correctly. The basal ganglia, cerebellum, and thalamus provide motor and sensory input about the planned speech movements. The limbic system and right hemisphere provide information about the emotional context of the intended utterance. All of this information needs to be integrated and processed so that an intended message can be transformed into a sequence of neural impulses that will contract the appropriate muscles at the correct times. The enormity of this task was illustrated by Darley et al. (1975) who calculated that for every second a person is talking, a total of 140,000 neuromuscular contractions and relaxations occur in the speech production muscles. The neurological "mechanism" thought to control this remarkable process is called the motor speech programmer.

The Motor Speech Programmer

The **motor speech programmer** is a neural network in the brain that sequences the motor movements needed to produce speech accurately. The motor speech programmer is thought to accomplish this by first analyzing the linguistic, motor, sensory, and emotional information of a planned speech act. It obtains this information through its many neural connections with the cognitive, language, emotional, and motor planning areas of the brain. It then sequences that information into a neural code that represents the muscular contractions needed to produce the phonemes, words, and phrases in the intended utterance. If that neural code is sequenced correctly and is received intact at the neuromuscular junction, the muscles will contract in the proper sequence, and the resulting speech will be produced fluently. Included in this neural code are the stress and intonational patterns that are used to convey the communicative intent of the speaker. Through the sensory information received by the motor speech programmer, the code also reflects the immediate circumstances of the oral-motor structures. For example, the speaker may be chewing gum and the neural code must be modified accordingly to ensure clear articulation of the utterance despite material in the mouth.

Although numerous writers have described the motor speech programmer (Darley et al., 1975; Duffy, 1995; and others), it is actually a rather indefinite, nebulous cerebral structure. Unlike Broca's and Wernicke's areas, the motor speech programmer has not been precisely localized in the brain. Research has indicated that it resides near the perisylvian area of the left hemisphere (Figure 11–1), where it has close

**Perisylvian Area of
the Left Hemisphere**

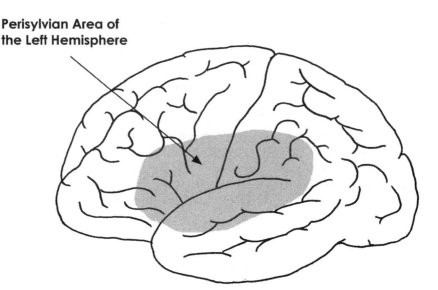

Figure 11–1. The perisylvian area of the left hemisphere. Damage to this area is often associated with instances of apraxia of speech.

associations with the language and motor centers of the brain. The motor speech programmer has especially close ties to Broca's area, which seems to play an important role in transforming the neural code into an accurate representation of the intended utterance (Brookshire, 1992). Even with clinical evidence such as this, the motor speech programmer remains a largely hypothetical entity. It is not too much of an exaggeration to say that its existence is inferred from only two facts: (a) humans have the ability to rapidly sequence speech movements and (b) damage to the left hemisphere can disrupt the ability to carry out this task. Further studies are needed to localize the motor speech programmer accurately and to more clearly understand how it accomplishes its complex operations.

ETIOLOGIES OF APRAXIA OF SPEECH

Disorders that damage the motor speech programmer have the potential to cause apraxia of speech. In practical terms, this means that apraxia of speech is the result of injury to the perisylvian area of the left hemisphere of the brain. Although damage to the left perisylvian area is the most common site of lesion in cases of apraxia of speech, it is not the only one. Injuries to the insula and the basal ganglia also have been associated with apraxia of speech. The specific conditions known to cause apraxia of speech include stroke, degenerative disease, trauma, and tumor. The most frequent cause of apraxia of speech is stroke. In a retrospective study at the Mayo Clinic, Duffy (1995) reported that strokes caused 58% of the cases of apraxia of speech over a 21-year period. Most of these strokes affected the perisylvian area of the left hemisphere, primarily the frontal and parietal lobes. Some cases of apraxia of speech also involved damage to the temporal lobe, but in each of these instances, frontal or parietal lobe damage was present as well.

The second most common cause of apraxia of speech in the Mayo study was degenerative disease, which accounted for 16% of the cases. These diseases included Alzheimer disease, primary progressive aphasia, and Creutzfeldt-Jakob disease. Although diseases such as these are usually associated with diffuse brain damage, Duffy (1995) indicated that at least in the early stages, their effects can be focal and result in apraxia of speech or other disorders associated with distinct lesions.

Trauma was the third most frequent cause of this disorder in the Mayo study, resulting in 15% of the cases. Surgical trauma in the left frontal lobe was the most common type of trauma that resulted in apraxia of speech. Aneurysm repair, removal of a tumor, and hemorrhage evacuation were some of the surgical procedures noted in the study. Although a few cases of closed head injury also resulted in apraxia of speech, most were the result of the more focal trauma of surgery.

The remaining 11% of the cases were caused by tumors in the left frontal lobe (6%), seizure disorder (1%), undetermined etiology (4%), or multiple causes (1%), such as a left hemisphere stroke and dementia. Duffy cautioned about generalizing the results of this retrospective study to the overall population because it was not a scientific sample of patients, but he also reported that the findings are in general agreement with those of a similar study by Wertz, Rosenbek, and Deal (1970).

SPEECH CHARACTERISTICS OF APRAXIA OF SPEECH

Studies of apraxia of speech have revealed many speech production errors that are unique to this disorder. Most researchers agree that apraxia of speech is a disorder primarily of articulation and prosody, although instrument-based studies have revealed problems in other areas of speech production, such as respiration. In general, individuals with this disorder are often described as having speech that is labored and halting. They may demonstrate instances of articulatory groping, which are trial-and-error attempts at finding the correct articulatory positions for target phonemes. Such groping may be especially noticeable at the beginning of an utterance or word. These individuals frequently will be inconsistent in their speech errors, perhaps making one error on a first attempt at a word and then making a different error on a second attempt. In severe cases of this disorder, the individuals may be nearly mute because they cannot voluntarily produce any sounds. Others with severe apraxia of speech may be only able to produce a few "stock" (stereotypic) phrases.

The following paragraphs present the specific characteristics of apraxia of speech. Of course, not all of these characteristics will be present in the speech of each individual with this disorder. There are several factors that influence how many aspects will be present. For example, the severity of the apraxia will influence how many of these characteristics may actually appear in a patient's speech (Miller, 1986). Individuals at the most severe and mild ranges of the disorder typically will demonstrate fewer examples of these characteristics than persons in the moderate range of severity. A co-occurring disorder, such as aphasia or dysarthria, also can affect how many of these characteristics will be present because the co-occurring conditions may mask the apraxic speech errors. An example of this could be when a patient has severe Broca aphasia and moderate apraxia of speech. The aphasia will restrict the patient's verbal expression so severely that few, if any, opportunities will arise for a demonstration of the apraxic speech errors.

Articulation

Without doubt, articulation errors are the most common problem in apraxia of speech. These errors arise from deficits in the patient's ability to smoothly sequence the oral movements needed to produce fluent speech. The following list of articulation errors that may be observed in individuals with apraxia of speech is a compilation of those reported by Darley et al. (1975), Duffy (1995), and Wertz et al. (1991). It is not a complete listing of errors, but it concentrates on the ones most likely to be encountered by the typical clinician and that can be most useful in making the diagnosis of apraxia of speech.

1. Substitutions of one phoneme for another are more common than distortions, omissions, additions, or repetitions. How-

ever, instrumentation or narrow transcription of these substitution errors often reveals that they are actually distortions of the target phoneme.

2. Placement errors are the most frequent type of substitution error, followed in order of commonality by manner, voicing, and oronasal errors.

3. The substitution of a voiceless phoneme for a voiced phoneme is more common than a substitution of a voiced phoneme for a voiceless.

4. Some substitution errors can be anticipatory (*llama* is pronounced "mama"), perseverative (*Viking* is pronounced "Viving"), or metathetic (*comfy chair* is pronounced "chumfy care").

5. Fricatives and affricates are generally more often in error than stops, nasals, semivowels, or vowels.

6. Consonant clusters are more likely to be in error than single consonants, and single consonants are more often in error than vowels.

7. The position of a phoneme within a word does not always determine whether it will be in error. When it does, however, phonemes in the initial position of a word are more likely to be in error than the medial or final position.

8. Phonemes that appear infrequently in speech are more often in error than frequently appearing phonemes.

9. Articulation is more accurate on real words compared to nonsense words.

10. Articulation errors are more common on multisyllabic words than single syllable words.

11. The farther the distance between the points of articulatory contact, the higher the rate of articulation errors. For example, "puh-tuh-kuh" is typically more difficult than "puh-puh-puh."

12. The voluntary production of speech (e.g., describing a picture) is more difficult than automatic speech (e.g., counting to 20) or reactive speech (e.g., swearing), although this may not always be true for individuals with severe apraxia of speech. As mentioned previously, these individuals may have apraxia to such a significant degree that they are nearly mute for all types of speech.

13. Articulation errors may be often quite inconsistent and can vary significantly during repeated utterances of the same word.

14. Sounds produced with the lips or with the tongue on the alveolar ridge are often easier to produce than sounds produced elsewhere.

Prosody

The prosody of individuals with apraxia of speech is frequently abnormal, but it is not exactly clear how apraxia affects prosody. Wertz et al. (1991), Duffy (1995), and others have offered several possibilities for how apraxia and prosody interact. One possibility is that prosody is disrupted by the patients' attempts to compensate for the articulatory errors in their speech. For example, the slow speech rate and equal syllable stress that is noted in apraxia of speech may be the result of patients purposely trying to maintain the best articulation possible while speaking. Second is the possibility that the many articulation deficits of this disorder make normal prosody extremely difficult. For instance, a patient who repeatedly stops an utterance, revises the articulation of a target sound, and then restarts the utterance will have great difficulty maintaining normal prosody. A final possibility for the interaction of apraxia and prosody is that prosodic errors are an integral part of apraxia of speech, just as the articulatory errors are. In other words, the prosodic errors in apraxia of speech are the direct result of a patient's motor sequencing deficit and not merely a reaction to it. Duffy (1995) indicated that instrumentation studies have provided some evidence for this third possibility, although the other two may be true as well. Wertz et al. (1991) concluded that, "prosodic disturbances probably reflect the effects of the primary motor deficit as well as the effort to compensate" (p. 69). The following is a list of the more obvious prosodic errors that may be present in patients with apraxia of speech.

1. The rate of connected speech is slower than normal.
2. Equal stress is often placed on all syllables in an utterance.
3. Silent pauses may occur at the initiation of a word or between syllables. These pauses may be the result of articulatory groping or because each syllable is being produced individually, instead of being produced with the normal fluent blending of one syllable into another.
4. The normal variations of pitch and loudness in utterances may be reduced.

Respiration

Apraxia has been shown to affect respiration. As mentioned previously, some individuals with apraxia of speech may not be able to voluntarily take a deep breath when asked to do so on command. When attempting this task, they will demonstrate the same halting, effortful movements seen in their articulation. Instrumentation has revealed more subtle respiration deficits in patients with apraxia. In a study of five subjects with apraxia, Keatley and Pike (1976) found that the amount of abnormal respiratory function was related to the severity of the subjects' apraxia of speech. The most severely affected subject demonstrated abnormal performance on 10 of the 13 measures of respiratory function. It is important to note, however, that these were voluntary respiratory tasks and that reflexive respiration is not affected by apraxia.

Resonance

Hyper- and hyponasality are seldom significant problems in apraxia of speech. Although there is little research into the velar movements of individuals with this disorder, the few studies that have been completed suggest that disturbed resonance in apraxia of speech seldom reaches the point where it is perceptible. For example, Itoh, Sasanuma, and Ushijima (1979) found that although velar movements can be inconsistent on repetitive movements, the general movement pattern of the velum usually remains within normal limits.

Phonation

Individuals with mild or moderate apraxia of speech seldom demonstrate isolated deficits of phonation. When they do have difficulties with phonation, it is usually in conjunction with an articulation problem. For example, there may be a delay in initiating the phonation of the first phoneme in a word, but this delay is part of the individual's groping for the correct articulatory position for that phoneme. In some cases of severe apraxia of speech, however, the patients will have significant deficits in their ability to phonate. For instance, they may be unable to complete such a "simple" phonatory task as prolonging a vowel. In these instances, the patients' motor speech sequencing is so disrupted that both voluntary and spontaneous attempts at phonation are unsuccessful. Duffy (1995) reported that such severe phonatory deficits usually occur in the first 1 or 2 weeks following the onset of the apraxia. If they continue beyond this period, such phonatory deficits usually indicate the presence of a co-occurring disorder, such as severe aphasia or akinetic mutism.

It is rare for a patient with apraxia of speech to have phonatory deficits that are more severe than accompanying articulatory problems. In those individuals with severe apraxia of speech who cannot prolong a vowel, it is very likely that they have co-occurring articulatory problems that are just as severe as their phonatory deficits. However, Marshall, Gandour, and Windsor (1988) described a remarkable patient who was an exception. Their patient had a left-hemisphere stroke following the repair of a cerebral aneurysm. The patient's resulting speech and language deficits did not resemble those of Broca aphasia, dysarthria, or apraxia of speech. Rather, he demonstrated the omission of syllables and words, and he had numerous stutteringlike dysfluencies. For example, when greeted by someone he had seen only once before, he said "Face mem [remember], not name mem [remember]." Eventually, it was determined that the patient had a laryngeal apraxia that prevented the normal integration of phonation with the other components of speech production, especially articulation. The accuracy of this diagnosis was confirmed when the patient was taught to use an electrolarynx. With this device providing the voicing for his speech, he communicated normally, using correct articulation, syntax, and grammatical morphemes.

DIFFERENTIAL DIAGNOSIS OF APRAXIA OF SPEECH

As mentioned, the errors in apraxia of speech are not caused by muscle weakness, abnormal muscle tone, reduced range of movement, or decreased muscle steadiness. This disorder is strictly a problem of motor sequencing. Before making the diagnosis of apraxia of speech, it is important to rule out other conditions that can cause movement difficulties similar to those seen in apraxia. Brookshire (1992) discussed four such conditions. The first is **muscle weakness**, which can produce slow, labored movements in affected body parts. Such effortful movements may sometimes resemble the movements of apraxia. The first step in making the differential diagnosis between weakness and apraxia is determining which movements are affected. When muscle weakness is the cause of the movement difficulty, *all* movements of the affected body part will reflect the weakness. However, in cases of apraxia, it is only the voluntary movements of the affected body part that will have the problem; automatic and spontaneous movements usually will be performed normally. In a case of true apraxia of speech, for example, the patient may be able to spontaneously produce a very clear "hello" when greeting a clinician at the beginning of a treatment session. But later, in the middle of the treatment session, the patient's voluntary attempts to say *hello* may be filled with distorted or substituted phonemes, revisions, or other apraxic errors. If the patient's articulation errors were the result of weakness, all attempts at saying *hello* would show evidence of the imprecise articulation.

Sensory loss is the second condition that needs be examined carefully before confirming a diagnosis of apraxia. Brookshire noted that sensory loss does not necessarily cause a movement disorder, but it can contribute to slowed or clumsy movement of an affected body part. For example, sensory loss in oral structures can contribute to imprecise articulation of speech sounds, as anyone who has had dental treatment numbing can attest. When there is sensory loss in suspected cases of apraxia, it is important for the clinician to determine whether the movement difficulties are caused by the sensory loss or the apraxia. As in cases of muscle weakness, Brookshire indicated that when sensory loss is contributing to a movement deficit, the problem will be present in both volitional and automatic actions. When caused by apraxia, it will be mostly present only in volitional actions.

A **comprehension deficit** is the third factor that must be ruled out in suspected cases of apraxia. The clinician needs to be sure that what appears to be an apraxic error is not actually the patient's inability to understand the instructions for the task. To determine whether the inability to complete the task is due to apraxia or poor comprehension, Brookshire suggested that the clinician demonstrate the target movement for the patient and ask questions about the movement, such as, "Am I drinking from a glass?" or "Am I rounding my lips?" If the answers to the questions are correct, the clinician can assume that the patient understands the task and has knowledge of what is represented by the movements. Any movement difficulties noted during the patient's subsequent attempts at the task can be presumed to be unrelated to a comprehension deficit.

Incoordination is the fourth condition that can sometimes be confused with the movement difficulties of apraxia. When individuals show signs of incoordination, such as in cases of cerebellar ataxia, they have movements that are slow and awkward. Although they usually do not have problems sequencing the individual steps of a movement, their clumsy movements sometimes mimic the halting, effortful movements seen in apraxia. To rule out incoordination in suspected cases of apraxia, Brookshire once again suggested that clinicians determine if the movement difficulty is present only in voluntary movements or if it is seen in all movements, both voluntary and automatic.

Differentiating Between Apraxia of Speech and Aphasia

In addition to distinguishing the errors of apraxia of speech from those of such conditions as muscle weakness, sensory loss, and so forth, clinicians often need to distinguish between apraxia of speech and aphasia. There are at least three situations in which clinicians may have difficulty making a differential diagnosis between these two disorders. The first is making a diagnosis between a patient with pure apraxia of speech and a patient either with aphasia alone or with aphasia *and* apraxia of speech. As mentioned at the beginning of this chapter, apraxia of speech can appear without any co-occurring aphasia. When it is present without aphasia, it is said to be pure apraxia of speech. Although pure apraxia of speech is quite rare, clinicians may encounter it occasionally. To determine if a patient has pure apraxia of speech or aphasia (either with or without an accompanying apraxia), it is important to remember that in pure apraxia of speech, the patient's auditory comprehension, reading, and writing will be largely unaffected by whatever caused the apraxia. This means that these three language modalities will be far more functional than the patient's verbal expression ability, which will demonstrate the articulation and prosody deficits of apraxia of speech. In contrast, aphasia will affect all four language modalities to one degree or another. The candidates for a diagnosis of pure apraxia of speech are patients who demonstrate the motor sequencing errors of apraxia of speech *and* have unaffected auditory comprehension, reading, and writing abilities. Only careful diagnostic testing of the patient's speech and language abilities will identify the patient with pure apraxia of speech.

The second situation that clinicians might find especially challenging is distinguishing between the errors of apraxia of speech and the literal paraphasic errors of aphasia. Literal paraphasic errors are the incorrect placement of one or more phoneme into a word. These errors most often are heard in individuals with fluent aphasia and, accordingly, are thought to be caused primarily by damage to Wernicke's area. In most instances, literal paraphasic errors consist of the transposition of phonemes or syllables in a word, the addition of extra phonemes to a syllable, or the substitutions of phoneme or syllables (Brookshire, 1992). At first glance, apraxia of speech and literal paraphasias can appear to be nearly identical because they both seem to involve the same type of phoneme-based errors. A closer examination, however, can reveal definite distinctions. Kent (1976) described a number of differences between apraxic errors and literal paraphasias.

1. Patients with apraxia of speech often have anterior brain damage and right hemiparesis. Patients with aphasia who produce literal paraphasias often have posterior brain damage and do not have hemiparesis.
2. Patients with apraxia of speech usually have a co-occurring Broca aphasia. Patients who produce literal paraphasias usually have Wernicke or conduction aphasia.
3. Patients with apraxia of speech usually have disturbed prosody, often because they are frequently stopping or slowing their speech as they grope for correct articulatory positions. Patients with aphasia usually produce their literal paraphasic errors in a flow of speech that has normal prosody.
4. Patients with apraxia of speech often have difficulty initiating speech, because they are searching for the correct articulatory position of the first word in an utterance. Patients with aphasia who produce literal paraphasias typically do not have as much trouble initiating an utterance.
5. The phoneme and syllable substitutions in apraxia of speech are usually close to the intended sounds. For example, a /b/ might be substituted for a /d/. The substitutions in literal paraphasias are often wildly off target from the intended sounds, such as a nasal consonant being used in place of a stop consonant, or perhaps even a vowel being substituted for a consonant.

If these distinctions are kept in mind, a thorough analysis of a patient's errors should reveal those that are apraxic and those that are literal paraphasias, at least in a majority of instances. But even the most knowledgeable clinician will not be able to identify every error correctly. It may be best to look primarily for a strong trend one way or the other when trying to determine whether a patient's phoneme-based errors are caused by apraxia or fluent aphasia.

The third challenging diagnostic situation is distinguishing apraxic speech errors from the nonfluent language errors of Broca aphasia. This can be an especially difficult task for several reasons. One is that there is little anatomical difference between sites of lesion for apraxia of speech and Broca aphasia. Although Broca area is not the exclusive site of lesion for either disorder, lower frontal lobe damage is frequently associated with both conditions. As a result, site of lesion information is usually not helpful in determining if a patient's errors are primarily caused by apraxia or Broca aphasia. Another reason it is difficult to tell these two disorders apart is that they co-occur so frequently. Most individuals with apraxia of speech also have Broca aphasia. This has led to the situation where the general descriptions of both disorders are often similar. Such words as nonfluent, effortful, halting, and disturbed prosody have been used to describe the speech of individuals with either disorder. Ultimately, it will be extremely difficult in many cases to tell precisely how many of a patient's errors are the result of apraxia or of Broca aphasia. The best a clinician can sometimes do is assess a patient's motor speech and language abilities as completely as possible and then make an estimate as to the severity of the apraxia in comparison to the Broca aphasia. If one condition is so severe as to mask the other, the clinician may want to take Rosenbek's (1978) advice that, "diagnosis of some patients with severe apraxia [and aphasia] may have to wait until the outcome of therapy is determined" (p. 193). In other words, it may be necessary to wait until treatment of the more obvious disorder reveals the hidden disorder.

KEY EVALUATION TASKS FOR APRAXIA OF SPEECH

1. One of the most sensitive assessments for apraxia of speech is the sequential motion rate (SMR) task, especially when compared to the patient's performance on the alternating motion rate (AMR) task. Many individuals with mild or moderate apraxia of speech can complete the AMR task accurately because it involves only one movement sequence with only one place of articulatory contact. However, they will be unable to complete the SMR task accurately because it requires the sequencing of multiple articulatory positions in three different sites within the mouth. The difference in their performance on these two tasks can be dramatic.
2. Conversational speech and reading are important tasks for determining the effects of the apraxia on prosody.
3. There are many other evaluation tasks that are sensitive to apraxia, such as repeating words of increasing length (e.g., *fan-fancy-fantastic*). These are included in the motor speech evaluation in Chapter 2.

TREATMENT OF APRAXIA OF SPEECH

Nearly all treatments for apraxia of speech are behaviorally based procedures that help affected individuals improve their ability to sequence speech sounds correctly. Unlike some of the treatments for dysarthria, prosthetic and medical interventions for apraxia of speech are rare. Most well-known treatments employ intensive one-on-one sessions in which the clinician and patient work on a sequence of tasks that progress from simple to complex verbal productions of target words and phrases. The treatment sessions for apraxia of speech tend to be time-intensive, repetitive, and highly structured. Because of this, the first impression of these treatments can be negative. However, there is a significant amount of evidence indicating that treatment for apraxia of speech can be effective, particularly if an accompanying aphasia is not too severe (Duffy, 1995). This section of the chapter examines the general concepts underlying apraxia treatment. It also presents the individual steps of several treatment programs. These steps are presented primarily to provide an idea of how the treatment sessions within a given program might be conducted. Readers are encouraged to seek out the original sources, if they are actually preparing to treat individuals with apraxia of speech. What is presented in this chapter are only summaries of the programs and are probably not detailed enough for direct clinical application.

General Principles

Darley et al. (1975) stated that the goal of treating apraxia of speech is to help the patient relearn the motor sequences needed to produce phonemes accurately. Most researchers who have studied apraxia treatment have described the general principles that are important in helping their subjects relearn speech movements. (Darley et al., 1975; Duffy, 1995; Rosenbek, Lemme, Ahern, Harris, & Wertz, 1973; Wertz et al., 1991). The similarity of these principles from writer to writer is striking. Their overall agreement suggests that there actually is a core set of factors that can facilitate the relearning of speech movements. This list is a collection of six such principles that seem to be essential to managing apraxia of speech.

> **1.** *Not all individuals with apraxia of speech are appropriate candidates for treatment.* Duffy (1995) indicated that some patients with severe aphasia and apraxia of speech may be too aphasic

to benefit from apraxia treatment. If a patient's language impairments are so severe that functional speech production is impossible, what will be the benefit of treating the apraxia? In this situation, it may be best to postpone the apraxia treatment until the patient's language abilities improve sufficiently to allow for better speech production. If the language abilities do not improve to this degree, apraxia treatment would not be appropriate for these individuals. Perhaps the treatment time would be better spent on continued language treatment or enhancing nonverbal communication skills through the use of gestures and augmentative communication devices.

2. *Patients and families need to understand the characteristics of apraxia and the rationale for the treatment tasks.* Wertz et al. (1991) stressed the importance of counseling patients and families about the nature of this disorder and the treatment process. They reported that it can be especially important to help patients and families understand the reasons behind the treatment tasks clinicians ask the patients to complete. For example, patients and families need to know why treatment usually begins with syllables or short words, why there is so much repetition, and why progress may be slow.

3. *Repetitive and intensive drillwork is an essential part of most treatment programs.* To relearn the motor sequences of intelligible speech, patients with apraxia of speech need to practice and rehearse the movements of speech production over and over again. The repetitive nature of this treatment is largely a consequence of the brain injury, in that individuals with such an injury typically need to work harder and longer to relearn a task (Rosenbek et al., 1973).

4. *The treatment should be sequenced carefully so that the patient is able to maintain a high success rate.* This means that patients begin with easy activities and only progress to more difficult ones when they are able to continue being accurate on the tasks. Wertz et al. (1991) said that the success rate in treatment could vary. For example, a typical patient will make many more errors in the very beginning of a treatment program than later, when they are more familiar with a task. In this situation, what constitutes an adequate success rate for the beginning of treatment will differ from what will be acceptable later in treatment.

5. *Patients should learn to monitor their own speech.* The importance of this is stressed by numerous writers (Duffy, 1995; Rosenbek et al., 1973; Wertz et al., 1991). It is a great asset for individuals with apraxia of speech to be able to listen for their own errors

and self-correct them. Feedback from the clinician can facilitate this ability in many patients. When the clinician gives information on what is an acceptable production of a target syllable, word, or phrase, patients are better able to judge what is correct or incorrect. It is not unusual, however, to find many patients who can make accurate judgments about their verbal productions without help from the clinician.

6. *Treatment should concentrate on functional and useful words as soon as possible.* Rosenbek et al. (1973) noted that because patients with apraxia of speech have lived most of their lives using verbal communication normally, it is important that they begin speaking meaningful words as early in a treatment sequence as possible. Although recognizing that some treatment needs to begin at the single phoneme level, Wertz et al. (1991) stated meaningful stimuli is more reinforcing than nonsense words and that it is easier for patients to judge the accuracy of their productions when real words are being spoken.

Specific Treatments

A number of specific treatments for apraxia of speech have been developed over the past 25 years. The following portion of this chapter describes several of these programs, all of which are published methods of managing apraxia of speech. To one degree or another, all of them incorporate the general principles of apraxia treatment mentioned in the previous paragraphs. The choice of which one to use with a given patient depends on several factors. One of the most important is the patient's preference. If a patient is not comfortable with the procedures in a treatment program or has doubts about a program's effectiveness, progress will probably be less than optimal. For example, there are some patients who will enjoy the melody-based drills in Melodic Intonation Therapy (MIT); there will be others who will not. Some patients will permit the clinician to perform the "hands on" manipulations of their oral structures as part of the PROMPT program; others will not. Determining a patient's preference is sometimes a trial-and-error process, and clinicians need to be willing to modify or drop a treatment procedure that is not working with a particular patient.

Another factor in choosing one of these techniques is the severity of the apraxia. Some programs seem to concentrate on the more severely involved patients (e.g., PROMPT, MIT); others might be appropriate for milder patients because of the ease with which certain steps can be skipped or modified (e.g., The Eight-Step Continuum). Familiarity with numerous treatment programs and procedures will facilitate the clinician's choice of which treatment to use with patients of different severity levels.

Lastly, the clinician's preference can be a factor in determining which program will be selected for use. All clinicians develop a predilection for certain treatment techniques. Sometimes this preference is based on what best suits an individual's clinical style; sometimes it is just the result of learning which is the more effective treatment procedure. Clinicians need to be convinced of their treatment's effectiveness, just as patients do. This knowledge of what works best is acquired partly by reading about the programs, partly by practical experience with them.

The Eight-Step Continuum Treatment

This treatment program was developed by Rosenbek et al. (1973). It is an eight-step sequence of structured activities that moves the patient from repeating target phonemes with the clinician to independent productions of utterances in role-playing situations. One of the key elements of this treatment is the careful selection of target sounds and words. The authors list five principles that will facilitate the patient's progression through the eight-steps.

- Begin with the easiest speech sounds and then move to the more difficult ones. Vowels, nasals, and stops are the easier sounds; fricatives, affricates, and consonant clusters are more difficult.
- As the patient begins to sequence sounds together, gradually increase the distance between points of articulatory contact in the target words. For example, the first target words or syllables may only contain bilabial consonants; the next may have both bilabials and lingua-alveolar sounds; the next may have bilabial and velar sounds.
- Choose the initial phonemes of target words carefully. Words that begin with vowels, nasals, or stops are more likely to be produced correctly than words beginning with fricatives, affricates, or consonant clusters.
- Gradually increase the length of the target words. It is best to start with short words that have repeating syllables, such as *B-B*, *so-so*, and *ta-ta*. Once these are mastered, systematically begin using longer words that have more complex syllable structure.

- When choosing real words for treatment, start with words that appear more often in day-to-day speech (i.e., high frequency words).

Once these principles are incorporated into the selection of initial target syllables or words, the treatment sequence is ready to begin. While guiding the patient through the eight treatment steps, the clinician should keep in mind several general rules: (a) move through the steps at a pace that keeps the patient successful; (b) repetitive drill will be necessary to help the patient relearn the motor sequences needed to produce volitional speech; (c) use functional, useful words in treatment as soon as possible; (d) encourage the patient to self-correct errors; and (e) teach compensatory strategies to facilitate speech, such as prolonging vowels, slowing rate, and pausing when needed.

The actual treatment steps in this program follow a logical sequence that moves from maximal to minimal cueing by the clinician. The following list is a summary of what the clinician and patient do in each of the eight steps. Of course, not all patients need to start on Step 1 or move through every step. Some will be able to skip steps, depending on the severity of their deficits.

1. The clinician tells the patient to "Watch me" and "Listen to me" and says the target word. They then both say the target word in unison.
2. The clinician tells the patient to "Watch me" and "Listen to me" and says the target word. Then, while the clinician silently mouths the word, the patient says the word aloud.
3. The clinician tells the patient to "Watch me" and "Listen to me" and says the target word. The patient then repeats the word independently.
4. The clinician tells the patient to "Watch me" and "Listen to me" and says the target word. The patient then repeats the word several times independently.
5. The clinician presents the target word written on paper, and the patient says the word while looking at it.
6. The clinician presents the target word written on paper, removes it, and then the patient says the word.
7. The patient says the word in response to a question from the clinician. For example, if the target word were the patient's name, the clinician would ask, "What is your name?" The patient would then say his or her name.
8. Role playing with the clinician, family, or friends is used to evoke the target word in an appropriate conversational context.

Darley, Aronson, and Brown's Procedure

Darley et al. (1975) described a direct approach to helping individuals with apraxia of speech relearn the motor sequences for speech production. It begins with a patient who is having difficulty with voluntary phonations, tongue protrusions, and other simple oral movements. Darley et al. called these beginning procedures "Initiating Speech Activities."

1. Encourage the patient to prolong an "ah." If this is not possible, see if the patient can voluntarily cough. If so, then try to shape the cough into a prolonged exhalation or sigh. If these are not successful, see if the patient can hum a familiar song or complete an automatic, open-ended phrase, such as "The sky is _____" or "Open the _____."
2. When a phonation is produced, the patient is asked to say that sound repeatedly, using different durations and levels of loudness. Then the patient should be encouraged to try shaping the phonation into several vowel sounds, such as "ee," "oh," "oo," and so forth.
3. Once vowels are being produced, the patient is asked to imitate the clinician's model of /m/. Darley et al. recommended using a mirror to facilitate the volitional closing of mouth for the /m/. When this consonant is produced, the patient is asked to begin forming syllables with /m/ in the initial position, such as *me, moe,* and *moo.*
4. Slightly more complicated production of CV syllables can be encouraged by having the patient alternate between syllables with open and closed vowels, such as *moe-me, moe-me, moe-me.* This also can be accomplished by using syllables that have /w/ in the initial position.

Once these tasks are accomplished, the patient should be ready for the next portion of this treatment program, which is called "Using Automatic Responses." For these tasks, it is assumed that the patient is able to produce some automatic phrases, such as counting or other overlearned word sequences. Darley et al. recommended that patients attempt to recite automatic responses so that they can regain the experience of producing speech easily. A list of recommended automatic responses is:

1. Counting from 1 to 10.
2. Reciting the days of the week or months of the year.

3. Common expressions such as "hello," "how are you?" "fine," "very well," "thank you," "I don't know," and so forth.
4. Well-known materials including nursery rhymes, phrases from television commercials, and the Lord's Prayer.
5. Singing well-known songs.

The next step, called "Phonemic Drill," is a return to working on volitional speech production. It is hoped by this stage that the patient is beginning to attempt some utterances spontaneously, although they may be filled with apraxic errors. Darley et al. recommended using the integral stimulation "watch and listen" method of presenting these phonemic drill tasks to the patient.

1. The first step is to choose an easy phoneme such as /m/. The patient is asked to hum the /m/ after the clinician demonstrates what to do.
2. Then the patient adds a series of vowels to the /m/, such as *my, moe, maw, moo, may,* and *me.* These words are practiced 10 to 20 times each.
3. These CV words are then doubled, so that *me* becomes *me-me* and *may* becomes *may-may.* The patient again practices saying these words 10 to 20 times each.
4. The next step is to add /m/ to the end of the CV words. For example, *mom, moom, meem* would be some of words created for this step.
5. The patient next begins saying actual words. Choose words that begin with /m/ and have other easy phonemes in them. Darley et al. suggested words such as *more, man, mine, moon, mare, mat, map,* and *mum.* As with all of these steps, the words are practiced at least 10 to 20 times each.
6. Producing two-word phrases is the next step. Both words in the phrases should begin with /m/. Examples of words for this step include *my mom, my mail, miss me, much more,* and *make me.*
7. Now the patient produces two-word phrases that end with /m/, such as *come home, name him, lame lamb, dumb bum,* and so forth.
8. The step has the patient say two-word phrases where /m/ is in the initial position of the first word and in the final position of the second. Examples would include *make him, my home, must name, my name, meet them,* and *Mary's room.*
9. The final step is having the patient produce longer phrases that include multisyllabic words, such as *moment by moment, my morning meeting, made much money, Monday morning,* and *among my memories.*

From here the patient moves to productions of other consonants in words, using the same sequence as with the /m/. Eventually, the patient will be asked to use the consonants he or she has mastered in words that contain the same vowel, such as *me, she, we, tea, bee, fee,* and *key*. Ultimately, the goal is to incorporate these words into phrases and then into sentences.

Melodic Intonation Therapy

Melodic Intonation Therapy (MIT) (Helm-Estabrooks, Nicholas, & Morgan, 1989) is based on the observation that many individuals with aphasia or apraxia of speech can sing the words of a song much better than they can say the same words in conversation. Many clinicians have worked with patients who could sing the words of a well-known song intelligibly, but when asked to say the words, they could not. One theory for this phenomenon is that singing is accessed through the undamaged right hemisphere. It is thought that singing the words of a song somehow allows the right hemisphere to facilitate the function of the damaged left hemisphere, resulting in better verbalizations in song than in conversation. MIT was designed to capitalize on this by blending rhythm and melody into the volitional speech of individuals with aphasia or apraxia of speech. In the MIT program, the rhythm and melody aspects of the program are emphasized primarily in the beginning steps of the program. The patient's intonation is then modified into a more natural prosody in the final steps.

The authors identified the patients who probably will be the most successful treatment candidates for this program. They reported that the best patients for MIT are those who (a) experienced a stroke, (b) have nonfluent aphasia or otherwise restricted verbal output, (c) have good auditory comprehension, (d) demonstrate poor articulation and repetition abilities, and (e) are motivated and have an adequate attention span. Patients with large lesions in Wernicke's area or have co-occurring right hemisphere damage are unlikely to benefit from the MIT program.

The MIT program is divided into three levels, with each level containing several individual steps. In the first two levels, the patient works on producing short, high-frequency words and phrases. The third level concentrates on longer, more complex utterances. The overall sequence of treatment is to first incorporate melodic intonation into the target utterances, then gradually shift to saying the words with exaggerated prosody, and finally saying the words with normal prosody. The following is a summary of the MIT treatment sequence.

Elementary Level

1. First the clinician demonstrates the melody by humming and singing the target word. The clinician taps the patient's hand on each syllable of the word or phrase. The patient does not respond, but only listens carefully.
2. The clinician and patient sing the target word and tap out the syllables together.
3. The clinician and patient begin by singing and tapping the word together, but the clinician stops about half way through. The patient is required to complete the word alone.
4. The clinician sings and taps the target first; the patient then repeats it immediately.
5. When the patient repeats the word from Step 4, the clinician immediately asks a question such as, "What did you say?" The patient attempts to say the target word in response to this question.

Intermediate Level

The four steps of this level follow the general sequence found in the prior level, except that delays of several seconds are inserted between the clinician's presentation of the target word and the patient's response. Length and complexity of the target words and phrases in this level are approximately the same as in the first level.

Advanced Level

The five steps in this portion of the program also concentrate on the delayed repetition of target phrases, as was done in the Intermediate Level. However, the melody used in the patient's utterances in the prior levels is now modified to match more closely normal speech intonation through a procedure called *speech-song*. The authors describe speech-song as being similar to choral reading, in that the rhythm and stress of the target phrase is exaggerated. The words are not actually sung in a melody. In the final step, the clinician asks a question, the patient waits about 6 seconds, and then answers with the correct target phrase using normal intonation.

Prompt

PROMPT is an acronym for Prompts for Restructuring Oral Muscular Targets. It was developed originally as a treatment for children with developmental apraxia of speech. The PROMPT program uses a combination of proprioceptive, pressure, and kinesthetic cues that show patients how to sequence their oral movements for speech (Square-Storer & Hayden, 1989). The clinician provides these cues by touching the patient's face and manually guiding the articulators to the appropriate positions needed to produce the target sounds. These "hands on" cues are designed to provide the patients with sensory information regarding place of articulatory contact, extent of jaw opening, voicing, relative timing of syllables, manner of articulation, and coarticulation. The basic premise of PROMPT is that clinicians are acting as external motor speech programmers when they are guiding the patient's articulators through the correct motor sequence to produce a target sound.

PROMPT identifies numerous contact points around the mouth, under the chin, and on the neck where clinicians place their fingers and hands to guide the articulators into the proper positions for speech production. The overall sequence of a PROMPT treatment is to first have the clinician say the target syllable, word, or phrase. The patient then attempts to say the word. If correct, the next word is presented. If incorrect, the clinician finds the correct contact points for the phonemes of the word and moves the patient's articulators passively. The patient is then asked to try saying the word again with the clinician simultaneously moving the articulators into the correct positions for the word's phonemes. Some of the cues are simple and can be understood by any clinician, such as those for bilabial sounds, voicing, and jaw opening. Many, however, are complex and require special instructions from a PROMPT workshop to understand fully. For example, the more dynamic cues, such as those for coarticulation or phrases, can be quite intricate. Nevertheless, PROMPT has been effective in helping some patients with co-occurring severe Broca's aphasia and apraxia of speech use a core vocabulary of a few words and phrases (Square, Chumpelik, & Adams, 1985; Square, Chumpelik, Morningstar, & Adams, 1986).

REVIEW OF APRAXIA OF SPEECH

- Apraxia of speech is a disorder of motor sequencing. It is not caused by muscle weakness, abnormal muscle tone, reduced range of movement, or decreased muscle steadiness.
- Apraxia of speech is a subcategory of ideomotor apraxia, which is defined as a disturbance in the performance needed to complete an action. This contrasts with ideational apraxia, which is a disturbance in the idea or purpose of a movement.

- The two most salient characteristics of ideomotor apraxia are (a) voluntary movements are affected more than spontaneous or automatic movements and (b) movement sequencing errors are often quite inconsistent from trial to trial.
- The neural network thought to control the sequencing of speech movements is called the motor speech programmer. It is an indistinct cerebral structure that seems to be located primarily in the left hemisphere of the brain.
- Apraxia of speech has numerous potential etiologies including stroke, degenerative diseases, trauma, and tumor.
- Apraxia of speech is primarily a disorder of articulation and prosody.
- When diagnosing apraxia of speech, it is important to eliminate conditions that can cause speech errors similar to those in apraxia of speech. Brookshire (1992) listed four such conditions: muscle weakness, sensory loss, comprehension deficit, and incoordination.
- Many treatments for apraxia of speech have been developed. The choice of which is best can depend on the severity of the apraxia and the patient's personal preferences.

STUDY QUESTIONS

1. Define apraxia of speech in your own words.
2. Describe how apraxia of speech is both similar and different from dysarthria.
3. How are ideational apraxia and ideomotor apraxia different?
4. Limb apraxia, nonverbal oral apraxia, and apraxia of speech are subcategories of which type of apraxia?
5. What is the difference between nonverbal oral apraxia and apraxia of speech?
6. What is the motor speech programmer?
7. The motor speech programmer receives input from what other parts of the brain?
8. What is the most common cause of apraxia of speech?
9. Why do patients with mild or severe apraxia of speech typically demonstrate fewer apraxic speech errors than patients with moderate apraxia of speech?
10. Apraxia of speech is primarily a disorder of which two components of speech production?
11. What are two of the possible ways in which apraxia of speech affects prosody?

12. When making the diagnosis of apraxia of speech, why must such conditions as weakness and reduced range of movement be eliminated as possible causes of a speech disorder?
13. Why can it be especially difficult to distinguish apraxia of speech from Broca aphasia?
14. What is one of the most sensitive evaluation tasks for identifying apraxia of speech?
15. What is integral stimulation?

References

Ackermann, H., & Ziegler, W. (1991). Cerebellar voice tremor: An acoustic analysis. *Journal of Neurology, Neurosurgery, and Psychiatry, 54,* 74–76.

Adams, S. G. (1994). Accelerating speech in a case of hypokinetic dysarthria: Descriptions and treatment. In J. A. Till, K. M. Yorkston, & D. R. Beukelman (Eds.), *Motor speech disorders: Advances in assessment and treatment* (pp. 213–228). Baltimore: Paul H. Brookes.

Adams, S. G. (1997). Hypokinetic dysarthria in Parkinson's disease. In M. R. McNeil (Ed.), *Clinical management of sensorimotor speech disorders* (pp. 261–286). New York, Thieme.

"Aphorisms of Hippocratic Corpus." (400 BC/1995). [CD-ROM]. *World's greatest classic books.* Salinas, CA: Corel.

Aronson, A. E. (1990). *Clinical voice disorders.* New York: Thieme.

Azrin, N. H., & Peterson, A. L. (1990). Treatment of Tourette's syndrome by habit reversal: A waiting-list control group comparison. *Behavior Therapy, 21,* 305–318.

Bergin, A., Waranch, H. R., Brown, J., Carson, K., & Singer, H. S. (1998). Relaxation therapy in Tourette syndrome: A pilot study. *Pediatric Neurology, 18,* 136–142.

Berry, W. R., Aronson, A. E., Darley, F. L., & Goldstein, N. P. (1974). Effects of penicillamine therapy and low-copper diet on dysarthria in Wilson's disease (hepatolenticular degeneration). *Mayo Clinic Proceedings, 49,* 405–408.

Berry, W. R., Darley, F. L., Aronson, A. E., & Goldstein, N. P. (1974). Dysarthria in Wilson's disease. *Journal of Speech and Hearing Research, 17,* 169–183.

Beukelman, D. R., Kraft, G., & Freal, J. (1985). Expressive communication disorders in persons with multiple sclerosis: A survey. *Archives of Physical Medicine and Rehabilitation, 66,* 675–677.

Beukelman, D. R., & Mirenda, P. (1998). *Augmentative and alternative communication* (2nd ed.). Baltimore: Paul H. Brooks.

Brodal, P. (1992). *The central nervous system: Structure and function.* New York: Oxford University Press.

Brookshire, R. H. (1992). *Introduction to neurogenic communication disorders* (4th ed.). St. Louis: Mosby.

Cannito, M. P., & Marquardt, T. P. (1997). Ataxic dysarthria. In M. R. McNeil (Ed.), *Clinical management of sensorimotor speech disorders* (pp. 217–248). New York: Thieme.

Canter, G. J. (1963). Speech characteristics of patients with Parkinson's disease: I. Intensity, pitch, and duration. *Journal of Speech and Hearing Disorders, 28,* 221–229.

Canter, G. J. (1965). Speech characteristics of patients with Parkinson's disease: III. Articulation, diadochokinesis, and over-all speech adequacy. *Journal of Speech and Hearing Disorders, 30,* 217–224.

Cole, M. F., & Cole, M. (1971). *Pierre Marie's papers on speech disorders.* New York: Hafner Publishing Company.

Dagenais, P. A., Southwood, M. H., & Lee, T. L. (1998). Rate reduction methods for improving speech intelligibility of dysarthric speakers with Parkinson's disease. *Journal of Medical Speech Language Pathology, 3,* 143–157.

Darley, F. L. (1969, November). *Aphasia: Input and output disturbances in speech and language processing.* Paper presented to the annual meeting of the American Speech-Language-Hearing Association, Chicago.

Darley, F. L. (1983). Foreword. In W. R. Berry (Ed.), *Clinical dysarthria* (pp. xiii–xv). San Diego: College-Hill Press.

Darley, F. L., Aronson, A. E., & Brown, J. R. (1969a). Clusters of deviant speech dimensions in the dysarthrias. *Journal of Speech and Hearing Research, 12,* 462–496.

Darley, F. L., Aronson, A. E., & Brown, J. R. (1969b). Differential diagnostic patterns of dysarthria. *Journal of Speech and Hearing Research, 12,* 246–269.

Darley, F. L., Aronson, A. E., & Brown, J. R. (1975). *Motor speech disorders.* Philadelphia: W. B. Saunders.

Darley, F. L., Aronson, A. E., & Goldstein, N. P. (1972). Dysarthria in multiple sclerosis. *Journal of Speech and Hearing Research, 15,* 229–245.

Downie, A. W., Low, J. M., & Lindsay, D. D. (1981). Speech disorders in parkinsonism: Usefulness of delayed auditory feedback in selected cases. *British Journal of Disorders of Communication, 16,* 135–139.

Duffy, J. R. (1995). *Motor speech disorders: Substrates, differential diagnosis, and management.* St. Louis: Mosby.

Duffy, J. R., & Folger, N. W. (1986, November). *Dysarthria in unilateral central nervous system lesions.* Paper presented at the annual meeting of the American Speech-Language-Hearing Association, Detroit, MI.

Dworkin, J. P. (1991). *Motor speech disorders: A treatment guide.* St Louis: Mosby.

Dworkin, J. P., & Johns, D. F. (1980). Management of velopharyngeal incompetence in dysarthria: A historical review. *Clinical Otolaryngology, 5,* 61–74.

Eggert, G. H. (1977). *Wernicke's works on aphasia: A sourcebook and review.* The Hague: Mouton Publishers.

Garrison, F. H. (1925/1969). History of neurology [revised and enlarged by L. C. McHenry, Jr.]. Springfield, IL: Charles C. Thomas.

Hardcastle, W. J., Barry, R. A., & Clark, C. J. (1985). Articulatory and voicing characteristics of adult dysarthric and verbal dyspraxic speakers: An instrumental study. *British Journal of Communication Disorders, 20,* 249–270.

Hartman, D. E., & Abbs, J. H. (1992). Dysarthria associated with focal unilateral upper motor neuron lesion. *European Journal of Disorders of Communication, 27,* 187–196.

Haynes, W. O., & Pindzola, R. H. (1998). *Diagnosis and evaluation in speech pathology* (5th ed.). Boston: Allyn & Bacon.

Heilman, K. M., Watson, R. T., & Greer, M. (1977). *Handbook for differential diagnosis of neurologic signs and symptoms.* New York: Appleton-Century-Crofts.

Helm-Estabrooks, N., Nicholas, M., & Morgan, A. R. (1989). *Melodic intonation therapy* (Manual). San Antonio, TX: Special Press, Inc.

Hirose, H. (1986). Pathophysiology of motor speech disorders (dysarthria). *Folia Phoniatria, 38,* 61–88.

Itoh, M., Sasanuma, S., & Ushijima, T. (1979). Velar movements during speech in a patient with apraxia of speech. *Brain and Language, 7,* 227–239.

Joanette, Y., & Dudley, J. G. (1980). Dysarthric symptomatology of Friedreich's ataxia. *Brain and Language, 10,* 39–50.

Johnson, J. A., & Pring, T. R. (1990). Speech therapy and Parkinson's disease: A review and further data. *British Journal of Disorders of Communication, 25,* 187–192.

Keatley, M. A., & Pike, P. (1976). An automated pulmonary function laboratory: Clinical use in determining respiratory variations in apraxia. In R. H. Brookshire (Ed.), *Clinical aphasiology: Conference proceedings.* Minneapolis, MN: BRK Publishers.

Kent, R. (1976). *Study of vocal tract characteristics of in the dysarthrias.* Presented to the Veterans Administration Workshop on Motor Speech Disorders, Madison, WI.

Kohen, D. P., & Botts, P. (1987). Relaxation-imagery (self-hypnosis) in Tourette syndrome: Experience with four children. *Journal of Clinical Hypnosis, 29,* 227–237.

Lechtenberg, R. (1982). *The psychiatrist's guide to diseases of the nervous system.* New York: John Wiley and Sons.

Lehiste, I. (1965). *Some acoustic characteristics of dysarthria speech; Bibliotheca phonetica: no. 2.* Basel, Switzerland: S. Karger.

Linebaugh, C. W. (1979). The dysarthrias of Shy-Drager syndrome. *Journal of Speech and Hearing Disorders, 44,* 55–60.

Linebaugh, C. W. (1983). Treatment of flaccid dysarthria. In W. H. Perkins (Ed.), *Current therapy in communication disorders: Dysarthria and apraxia.* New York: Thieme.

Logemann, J. A., Fisher, H. B., Boshes, B., & Blonsky, E. R. (1978). Frequency and cooccurrence of vocal tract dysfunctions in the speech of a large sample of Parkinson patients. *Journal of Speech and Hearing Disorders, 43,* 47–57.

Luchsinger, R., & Arnold, G. E. (1965). *Voice-speech-language* (G. E. Arnold & E. R. Finkbeiner, Trans.). Belmont, CA: Wadsworth Publishing Company, Inc.

Ludlow, C. L., & Bassich, C. J. (1984). Relationships between perceptual ratings and acoustic measures of hypokinetic speech. In M. R. McNeil, J. C. Rosenbek, & A. E. Aronson (Eds.), *The dysarthrias: Physiology, acoustics, perceptions, management* (pp. 163–196). San Diego: College-Hill Press.

Ludlow, C. L., Conner, N. P., & Bassich, C. J. (1987). Speech timing in Parkinson's and Huntington's disease. *Brain and Language, 32,* 195–214.

Luria, A. (1972). *The man with a shattered world.* Harmindsworth: Penguin.

Mahler, S. M., Luke, J. A., & Daltroff, W. (1945). Clinical and follow-up study of the tic syndrome in children. *American Journal of Orthopsychiatry, 15,* 631–647.

Marshall, R. C., Gandour, J., & Windsor, J. (1988). Selective impairment of phonation: A case study. *Brain and Language, 35,* 313–339.

Miller, N. (1986). *Dyspraxia and its management.* Rockville, MD: Aspen Publishers.

Moore, C. A., Yorkston, K. M., & Beukelman, D. R. (Eds.). (1991). *Dysarthria and apraxia of speech: Perspectives on management.* Baltimore: Paul H. Brookes.

Murdoch, B. E., Chenery, H., Stokes, P., & Hardcastle, W. (1991). Respiratory kinematics in speakers with cerebellar disease. *Journal of Speech and Hearing Research, 34,* 768–780.

Murdoch, B. E., Thompson, E. C., & Theodoros, D. G. (1997). In M. R. McNeil (Ed.), *Clinical management of sensorimotor speech disorders* (pp. 287–310). New York: Thieme.

Netsell, R., & Kent, R. (1976). Paroxymal ataxic dysarthria. *Journal of Speech and Hearing Disorders, 41,* 93–109.

Nicolosi, L., Harryman, E., & Kresheck, J. (1983). *Terminology of communication disorders: Speech-language-hearing* (2nd ed.). Baltimore: Williams and Wilkins.

"Of the epidemics of Hippocratic Corpus." (400 BC/1995). [CD-ROM]. *World's Greatest Classic Books.* Salinas, CA: Corel.

O'Neill, Y. V. (1980). *Speech and speech disorders in western thought before 1600.* Westport, CT: Greenwood Press.

Parker, H. L. (1969). *Clinical studies in neurology.* Springfield, IL: Charles C. Thomas.

Peterson, B. S., & Cohen, D. J. (1998). The treatment of Tourette's syndrome: Multimodal, developmental intervention. *Journal of Clinical Psychiatry, 59*(Suppl. 1), 62–72.

Przedborski, S., Brunko, E., Hubert, M., Mavroudakis, N., & de Beyl, D. Z. (1988). The effect of acute hemiplegia on intercostal muscle activity. *Neurology, 38,* 1882–1884.

Robin, D. A., Yorkston, K. M., & Beukelman, D. R. (Eds.). (1996). *Disorders of motor speech: Assessment, treatment, and clinical characterization.* Baltimore: Paul H. Brookes.

Ropper, A. H. (1987). Severe dysarthria with right hemisphere stroke. *Neurology, 37,* 1061–1063.

Rosenbek, J. C. (1978). Treating apraxia of speech. In D. F. Johns (Ed.), *Clinical management of neurogenic communicative disorders* (pp. 191–242). Boston: Little, Brown.

Rosenbek, J. C., & LaPointe, L. L. (1985). The dysarthrias: Description, diagnosis, and treatment. In D. F. Johns (Ed.), *Clinical management of neruogenic communication disorders* (pp. 251–310). Boston: Little, Brown.

Rosenbek, J. C., LaPointe, L. L., & Wertz, R. T. (1989). *Aphasia: A clinical approach.* Boston: College-Hill Press.

Rosenbek, J. C., Lemme, M. L., Ahern, M. B., Harris, E. H., & Wertz, R. T. (1973). A treatment for apraxia of speech. *Journal of Speech and Hearing Disorders, 38*, 462–472.

Rubow, R., & Swift, E. (1985). A microcomputer-based wearable biofeedback device to improve transfer of treatment in parkinsonian dysarthria. *Journal of Speech and Hearing Disorders, 50*, 178–185.

Saunders, C., Walsh, T., & Smith, M. (1981). Hospice care in the motor neuron diseases. In C. Saunders & J. Teller (Eds.), *Hospice: The living idea*. London: Edward Arnold.

Scott, S., & Caird, F. I. (1983). Speech therapy for Parkinson's disease. *Journal of Neurology, Neurosurgery, and Psychiatry, 46*, 140–144.

Smith, W. D. (1994). *Hippocrates: Volume VII*. Cambridge, MA: Harvard University Press.

Square, P., Chumpelik, D., & Adams, S. (1985). Efficacy of the PROMPT system of therapy for the treatment of acquired apraxia of speech. In R. Brookshire (Ed.), *Clinical aphasiology conference proceedings* (pp. 319–320). Minneapolis: BRK Publishers.

Square, P., Chumpelik, D., Morningstar, D., & Adams, S. (1986). Efficacy of the PROMPT system of therapy for the treatment of acquired apraxia of speech: A follow-up investigation. In R. Brookshire (Ed.), *Clinical aphasiology conference proceedings* (pp. 221–226), Minneapolis: BRK Publishers.

Square-Storer, P., & Hayden, D. (1989). PROMPT treatment. In P. Square-Storer (Ed.), *Acquired apraxia of speech in aphasic adults* (pp. 165–189). London: Taylor & Frances.

Swigert, N. B. (1997). *The source for dysarthria*. East Moline, IL: LinguiSystems, Inc.

Warlow, C. (1991). *Handbook of neurology*. Oxford: Blackwell Scientific Publications.

Wertz, R. T., LaPointe, L. L., & Rosenbek, J. C. (1991). *Apraxia of speech in adults: The disorder and its management*. San Diego: Singular Publishing Group.

Wertz, R. T., Rosenbek, J. C., Deal, J. L. (1970, November). *A review of 228 cases of apraxia of speech: Classification, etiology, and localization*. Paper presented to the American Speech-Language-Hearing Association, New York, NY.

Wiederholt, W. C. (1995). *Neurology for non-neurologists*. Philadelphia: W. B. Saunders Company.

Yorkston, K. M., Beukelman, D. R., & Bell, K. (1988). *Clinical management of dysarthric speakers*. San Diego: College-Hill Press.

Zraick, R. I., & LaPointe, L. L. (1997). Hyperkinetic dysarthria. In M. R. McNeil (Ed.), *Clinical management of sensorimotor speech disorders* (pp. 249–260). New York: Thieme.

Glossary

abduction Moving away from the midline, such as in abduction of the vocal folds.

acetylcholine Neurotransmitter at several sites in the nervous system, including at the neuromuscular junction and in the basal ganglia.

action tremor Tremor that is present only when an affected body part is being moved actively, such as when an arm and hand are outstretched. When the body part is at rest, the tremor is absent or greatly reduced in intensity.

adduction Moving toward the midline, such as in the adduction of the vocal folds.

afferent Neurons that convey neural impulses from the periphery to the central nervous system.

akinesia Delay in the initiation of movements; one of the most common characteristics of parkinsonism.

alternate motion rate (AMR) Rapid repetition of a single movement; usually obtained by timing patients as they repeat a syllable ("puh, puh, puh") as quickly, evenly, and clearly as possible.

amyotrophic lateral sclerosis (ALS) Degenerative neurological disease that ultimately affects upper and lower motor neurons; cognition retains intact as the disease progresses.

anatomy Study of the parts of the body and how the parts are related in structure.

aneurysm "Ballooning" of a blood vessel at a point of weakness; aneurysms are subject to rupture.

anoxia A lack of oxygen to tissue.

anterior In the front or forward part.

aphasia Acquired language deficit that affects verbal production, auditory comprehension, reading, and writing.

aphonia Loss or absence of voice.

apraxia Deficit in the ability to sequence the movements needed to carry out a familiar action.

apraxia, ideational Inability to use an object or gesture because the individual has lost the knowledge of the object's or gesture's function.

apraxia, ideomotor Disturbance in the ability to sequence the movements needed to use an object or perform a gesture; in contrast to ideational apraxia, the individual retains knowledge of the object's or gesture's function.

apraxia, limb Deficit in the ability to sequence familiar movement of the limbs; a subcategory of ideomotor apraxia.

apraxia, nonverbal oral Deficit in the ability to sequence oral movements that are not related to speech production.

apraxia of speech Deficit in the ability to sequence the movements of the articulators, resulting mainly in problems of articulation and prosody.

articulation Movement of the speech mechanism for the production of phonemes, syllables, and words.

articulators Components of the speech mechanism, usually said to be the lips, tongue, jaw, and velum; however, the vocal folds also can be considered to be one of the articulators in that they are used to produce /h/, which is often described as a glottal fricative phoneme.

association cortex Portions of the cerebral cortex that interpret and integrate sensory information from the primary cortex.

ataxia Deficits in the timing, force, range, and direction of voluntary movement; ataxia is caused by damage to the cerebellum or its control circuits.

axon Single long extension of a neuron that conducts neural impulses away from the cell body.

basal ganglia Collection of subcortical gray matter structures that play an important role in the refinement of movements.

bilateral Pertaining to both sides of an anatomical structure.

boutons, terminal Small projections at the end of an axon, which make synaptic connections with muscles, organs, glands, or other neurons.

bradykinesia Neurological deficit that results in movements that are slow and have reduced range of motion; often seen in parkinsonism.

brainstem Portion of the brain that connects the cerebral hemispheres with the spinal cord. It consists of the midbrain, pons, and medulla.

bulbar Pertaining to the brainstem, in particular to the medulla.

central nervous system (CNS) Brain and spinal cord.

cerebellar peduncles Three bundles of neural tracts that connect the cerebellum with the rest of the central nervous system.

cerebellum Part of the brain that is attached to the back of the brainstem and is responsible for coordinating movements.

cerebral cortex Outermost layer of the cerebrum.

cerebrovascular accident (CVA) Interruption of blood flow to the brain; also known as a stroke.

chorea Hyperkinetic movement disorder that results in involuntary movements that often are "dancelike" in appearance and usually affects many parts of the body, including the head, limbs, and torso.

collateral Small branch from an axon that enables a neuron to transmit its impulses to neurons not normally reached directly by the axon.

contralateral Pertaining to the opposite side.

coronal section Dividing a body part into front and back halves.

cortex External layer, usually used to describe the surface of the cerebrum.

corticobulbar tract Tract of upper motor neurons that course from the cortex to the brainstem; one of the tracts in the pyramidal system; it carries primarily motor impulses for skilled, voluntary movements.

corticospinal tract Tract of upper motor neurons that course from the cortex to the spinal cord; one of the tracts in the pyramidal system; it carries primarily motor impulses for skilled, voluntary movements.

cranial nerve nuclei Sites in the brainstem where the cell bodies of lower motor neurons in the cranial nerves are located.

cranial nerves Twelve pairs of nerves that branch from the brain; mostly from the brainstem.

decussation of the pyramids Place in the medulla where most axons in the corticospinal tract cross to the contralateral side of the body.

delayed auditory feedback (DAF) Electronic biofeedback effect, in which a device delays individuals' perception of their speech; sometimes used to slow the rate of speech in individuals with parkinsonism.

dendrites Short extensions from the neuron cell body that receive impulses from other neurons.

diplophonia Simultaneous phonation of two sounds, usually the result of hyperadducted vocal folds that cause vibrations in the false and true vocal folds.

direct activation system Another name for the pyramidal system.

dopamine Important neurotransmitter in the central nervous system, with considerable localization in the basal ganglia.

dorsal Pertaining to the back.

dysarthria Impaired production of speech because of disturbances in the neuromuscular control of the speech mechanism.

dyskinesia, tardive Delayed appearance of choreic movements after prolonged ingestion of certain neuroleptic (antipsychotic) drugs.

dystonia A hyperkinetic movement disorder that causes sustained involuntary contractions of muscle groups, body parts, or large areas of the body.

efferent Neurons that convey neural impulses from the central nervous system to the periphery.

equal and excess stress Equalization of stress that typically is variable in normal speech and placement of excessive stress on words or syllables that are typically unstressed.

extrapyramidal system Complex collection of upper motor neuron tracts that are "extra" to the pyramidal system; These tracts are responsible for controlling posture, reflexes, and muscle tone.

fasciculations Small spontaneous contractions of muscle tissue, often seen following lower motor neuron damage.

final common pathway Another name for lower motor neurons; so named because there is no further pyramidal or extrapyramidal influence on a motor impulse once it has started traveling along a lower motor neuron.

flaccid Weak or soft.

frontal Pertaining to the forehead; also located in the front.

ganglion Collection of neuron cell bodies in the peripheral nervous system; also small cystic tumors.

glottal stop Stop sound that is produced by the rapid release of subglottic air pressure at the vocal folds.

glottis Space between the true vocal folds.

gray matter Neural tissue that is rich with neuron cell bodies, which are gray in color.

Guillain-Barré syndrome Peripheral neuropathy that causes the acute inflammation of the myelin sheath around axons; also known as acute ideopathic polyneuritis.

gyrus Convoluted ridge on the surface of the brain; in contrast to a "groove" on the surface of the brain (sulcus).

gyrus, postcentral Another name for the primary sensory cortex.

gyrus, precentral Another name for the primary motor cortex.

hemiballism Violent motor movements of one side of the body; caused by damage to the subthalamic nucleus.

Hippocrates Greek physician; called historic father of modern medicine.

Hippocratic Corpus Collection of Greek medical texts probably written in the Fourth and Fifth centuries BC.

hyper- Prefix: excessive; above; more than normal.

hyperkinetic Class of movement disorders characterized by excessive, involuntary movements.

hypernasal Speech with excessive amounts of nasal resonance on nonnasal phonemes.

hypo- Prefix: too little; below; less than normal.

hypokinetic Class of movement disorders characterized by reduced and restricted movements; seen commonly in parkinsonism.

hyponasal Speech with too little nasal resonance on nasal phonemes.

ideational apraxia Inability to use an object or gesture because the individual has lost the knowledge of the object's or gesture's function.

ideomotor apraxia Disturbance in performance of the movements needed to use an object or gesture. In contrast to ideational apraxia, the individual retains knowledge of the object's or gesture's function.

idiopathic Spontaneous occurrence of a pathological condition with an unknown or obscure cause.

indirect activation system Another name for the extrapyramidal system.

inhalatory stridor Phonation on inhalation caused by the incomplete abduction of one or both vocal folds.

innervation Supply of nerve fibers functionally linked with a body part.

innervation ratio Relative number of muscle fibers innervated by one axon; a low innervation ratio (e.g., 25 fibers innervated by one axon) is seen in body parts that perform fine, skilled movements.

instrumental analysis Use of electronic or computerized instruments in the analysis of disorders, including motor speech disorders.

intention tremor Tremor that becomes more evident as the affected body part approaches a target, such as in reaching for an object.

internal capsule Subcortical site in the cerebrum where descending upper motor neurons are squeezed together as they pass between the thalamus and the basal ganglia.

interneurons Neurons that are between two other neurons; they often play a role in mediating communication between the two other neurons.

intonation Changes in pitch and stress that have communicative intent, such as the rising intonation of a question or the drop in intonation at the end of a statement.

ipsilateral Pertaining to the same side.

L-dopa A chemical precursor of dopamine; used to treat the effects of parkinsonism.

limb apraxia Deficit in the ability to sequence familiar movements of the limbs.

limbic system Collection of interconnected structures in the brain that helps control emotions.

lobe Well-defined area of an organ.

lower motor neuron Neuron in the cranial and spinal nerves that transmits motor impulses to muscles, organs, or glands; also known as the final common pathway.

mandible Jaw.

medial Pertaining to the midline or middle.

meninges Three membranes that cover the brain and spinal cord, namely the dura mater, arachnoid, and pia mater.

monoloudness Reduced vocal loudness variation during speech.

monopitch Reduced vocal pitch variation during speech.

motor neuron Neuron that transmits motor impulses.

motor speech disorders Collection of speech production deficits caused by the abnormal functioning of the motor system.

motor speech programmer Neural "mechanism" in the language-dominant hemisphere of the brain that creates the motor code needed to smoothly sequence and perform the complex movements of speech production; the motor speech programmer is an as yet ill-defined neurological structure.

motor strip Another name for the primary motor cortex or the precentral gyrus.

motor system Portion of the nervous system responsible for voluntary and involuntary body movements.

myasthenia gravis Disease that causes the destruction of acetylcholine receptors in muscle tissue, resulting in the rapid fatigue of muscle contractions.

myelin White, fatty covering around axons; myelin acts as insulation.

myo- Prefix: pertaining to muscle tissue.

nasal emission Audible or measurable escape of air through the nasal cavity during the production of nonnasal phonemes, usually most evident on voiceless stop and fricative consonants.

nerve Bundle of neurons in the peripheral nervous system; nerves carry impulses between the central nervous system and some other part of the body.

nerves, cranial Twelve pairs of nerves that branch from the brain, mostly from the brainstem.

nerves, spinal Thirty-one pairs of nerves that branch from the spinal cord. Spinal nerves innervate most of the body's muscles.

neural tract Bundle of neurons in the central nervous system; neurons in a neural tract convey similar types of impulses; this contrasts with nerves, which often carry both sensory and motor impulses.

neuroleptic Pertaining to the effects of antipsychotic drugs on cognition and behavior.

neurology Study of the nervous system and the disorders associated with the nervous system.

neuromuscular junction Place where the axons of lower motor neurons make synaptic connections with muscle tissue.

neuron Nervous system cell that can conduct and transmit electrochemical impulses.

neuron, lower motor Neuron in the cranial and spinal nerves that transmits motor impulses to muscles, organs, or glands.

neuron, motor Neuron that transmits motor impulses.

neuron, sensory Neuron that transmits sensory impulses through the nervous system.

neuron, upper motor Neuron in the central nervous system that ultimately makes synaptic connections with the lower motor neurons of the cranial and spinal nerves; the neurons of the pyramidal and extrapyramidal systems are upper motor neurons.

neurotransmitters Chemical released by the terminal boutons of an axon that either excite or inhibit the firing of an adjoining neuron.

nonverbal oral apraxia Deficit in the ability to sequence oral movements that are not related to speech production.

overarticulation Purposeful, exaggerated articulation of consonant phonemes; can often improve the intelligibility in dysarthric speakers.

pacing board Device that has numerous finger-width grooves along its length; sometimes can be used to slow the rate of speech of individuals with hypokinetic dysarthria.

palatal lift Intraoral prosthetic device that is attached to a dental retainer to facilitate the elevation of the velum during speech; used to treat incomplete velopharyngeal closure.

palsy Paralysis; also unchecked tremor.

parkinsonism Collection of neurological disorders with symptoms of tremor, bradykinesia, akinesia, muscle rigidity, and disturbed postural reflexes.

pathway, final common Another name for lower motor neurons; so named because there is no further pyramidal or extrapyramidal influence on a motor impulse once it has started traveling along a lower motor neuron.

perceptual analysis Use of a clinician's perceptions to analyze and evaluate motor speech disorders.

peri- Prefix: around; near.

peripheral nervous system (PNS) Cranial and spinal nerves.

perisylvian area Area around the Sylvian fissure of the brain.

pharyngeal flap procedure Surgical attachment of a flap of tissue from the pharynx to the velum; used to treat incomplete velopharyngeal closure.

phonation Production of acoustic energy by the vibration of the vocal folds.

physiology Study of the function of the parts of a living organism.

polio Acute viral infection that attacks the cell bodies of lower motor neurons.

postcentral gyrus Another name for the primary sensory cortex.

postural reflexes Reflexive movements that allow for the normal execution of such movements as walking, rising from a chair, or reaching for an object; the swinging of the arms while walking is an example of a postural reflex.

precentral gyrus Another name for the primary motor cortex.

premotor area Area of the frontal lobe that plays a role in the refinement of movements; the premotor area is especially important in controlling visually guided movements.

primary cortex Areas of the cerebral cortex that first receive sensory impulses from the body; however, the primary motor cortex is an exception; the primary motor cortex receives planned movements from cortical and subcortical areas of the brain.

prosody Melody of speech, which conveys meaning within an utterance through the use of intonation and stress.

pseudobulbar Condition whose symptoms mimic those seen after damage to the brainstem but is actually caused by another factor.

pseudobulbar affect Uncontrolled laughing or crying that occurs independently of the emotions actually felt by an individual; among motor speech disorders, it is most common in spastic dysarthria.

pyramidal system Upper motor neuron pathways that convey motor impulses for skilled, voluntary movements; the pyramidal system is divided into the corticobulbar and corticospinal tracts.

range of movement Distance that a body part can move when its muscles are contracted.

reflex Rapid, involuntary action in response to a stimulus.

resonance Placement of oral or nasal tonality onto phonemes during speech.

respiration "Power supply" of speech production; respiration provides the subglottic air pressure that is turned into acoustic energy by the speech production mechanism.

resting tremor Tremor that occurs when the affected body part is still; the tremor will typically disappear when the body part is actively being moved; resting tremor is common in parkinsonism.

reticular formation Specialized, complex collection of neurons in the brainstem that regulates arousal, respiration, and blood pressure; through its connections with the extrapyramidal system, the reticular formation plays an important role in postural reflexes.

rigidity Abnormal increase in muscle tone. Rigidity differs from spasticity in that the increased muscle tone is always constant. In spasticity, there is increasing and decreasing amounts of muscle tone as the affected body part is moved passively.

scanning speech Term often used by medical doctors to describe the slow and deliberate production of syllables and words in cases of ataxic dysarthria.

sensory neurons Neurons that transmit sensory impulses through the nervous system.

sensory strip Another name for the primary sensory cortex or the postcentral gyrus.

sensory tricks Idiosyncratic actions that individuals with dystonia employ to temporarily inhibit the involuntary muscular contractions of that disorder; examples include touching the chin to stop a focal mandibular dystonia or holding a piece of candy in the mouth to suppress a focal tongue dystonia.

sequential motion rate (SMR) Rapid repetition of a sequence of movements; usually obtained by timing patients as they repeat syllables ("puh, tuh, kuh") as quickly, evenly, and clearly as possible.

spasticity Abnormal increase in muscle tone. Spasticity differs from rigidity, in that the increased muscle tone is inconsistent as an affected body is moved passively. Initially, there will be an increase in muscle tone during a passive movement, but it can then disappear completely as the movement continues. In rigidity, the increased muscle tone is constant throughout all movements.

spinal nerves Thirty-one pairs of nerves that branch from the spinal cord. Spinal nerves innervate most of the body's muscles.

stress Changes in the pitch, loudness, and duration of syllables that give a word added importance or to clarify meaning.

stress, equal and excess Equalization of stress that is variable in normal speech and placement of excessive stress on words or syllables that are typically unstressed.

striatum Part of the basal ganglia, composed of the putamen and caudate nucleus.

substantia nigra Subcortical gray matter structure whose neurons provide the neurotransmitter dopamine to the striatum; the degeneration of these neurons causes the symptoms of idiopathic Parkinson's disease.

sulcus Groove in the surface of the brain.

supplementary motor area Area of the brain's frontal lobe that is important in the refining of motor movements, especially in movements that require complex actions of both hands.

synaptic cleft Microscopic gap between the terminal boutons of an axon and the dendrites of an adjoining neuron.

tardive dyskinesia Delayed appearance of choreic movements after prolonged ingestion of certain neuroleptic (antipsychotic) drugs.

Teflon injection Injection of Teflon into the posterior pharyngeal wall to create a small bulge, which lessens the distance the velum must travel before velopharyngeal closure is made.

terminal boutons Small projections at the end of an axon that make synaptic connections with muscles, organs, glands, or other neurons.

terminal ramifications Same as terminal boutons.

thalamus Subcortical gray matter structure through which all sensory information passes as it travels to the cortex and other areas of the brain; the thalamus plays a poorly understood role in the refinement of planned movements.

tic Involuntary, compulsive movement that is properly coordinated, such as eyeblinks and shoulder shrugs. Unlike other hyperkinetic movement disorders, tics are unique in that they can be suppressed voluntarily for a period.

tremor Involuntary, repetitive quivering of a body part.

tremor, action Tremor that is present only when an affected body part is being moved actively, such as when an arm and hand are outstretched; when the body part is at rest, the tremor is absent or greatly reduced in intensity.

tremor, intention Tremor that becomes more evident as the affected body part approaches a target, such as reaching for an object; common in cerebellar ataxia.

tremor, resting Tremor that occurs when the affected body part is still; the tremor will typically disappear when the body part is actively being moved; resting tremor is common in parkinsonism.

tumor Uncontrolled and progressive growth of tissue as a result of cell multiplication.

unilateral Pertaining to one side.

upper motor neuron Neuron in the central nervous system that ultimately makes synaptic connections with the lower motor neurons of the cranial and spinal nerves. The neurons that make up the pyramidal and extrapyramidal systems are upper motor neurons.

velopharyngeal incompetence Incomplete closure of the velopharyngeal port, usually resulting in hypernasal resonance.

ventral Pertaining to the front.

vital capacity Total air that can be exhaled from the lungs after a full inhalation.

white matter Myelin covered axons that course through the central nervous system; so named because myelin is white in color.

Wilson's disease Condition marked by the inability to metabolize dietary copper, which is deposited in the cornea of the eye, the brain, and other organs; Wilson's disease most often results in a mixed dysarthria.

Index